KU-200-606

MILADY
SalonOvations

BRAIDS & UPDO'S MADE EASY

WITHDRAWN

Delmar Publishers' Online Services

To access Delmar on the World Wide Web, point your browser to: **http://www.delmar.com/delmar.html**
To access through Gopher: **gopher://gopher.delmar.com**

(Delmar Online is part of "thomson.com", an Internet site with information on more than 30 publishers
of the International Thomson Publishing organization.)

For information on our products and services:

email: info@delmar.com   or   call **800-347-7707**

THE LIBRARY
GUILDFORD COLLEGE
of Further and Higher Education

SalonOvations'
BRAIDS & UPDO'S
MADE EASY

by Jamie Rines Jones

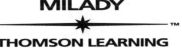
MILADY
★
™
THOMSON LEARNING

Africa • Australia • Canada • Denmark • Japan • Mexico • New Zealand • Philippines
Puerto Rico • Singapore • Spain • United Kingdom • United States

646.724 JON
151445

NOTICE TO THE READER

Publisher does not warrant or guarantee any of the products described herein or perform any independent analysis in connection with any of the product information contained herein. Publisher does not assume, and expressly disclaims, any obligation to obtain and include information other than that provided to it by the manufacturer.

The reader is expressly warned to consider and adopt all safety precautions that might be indicated by the activities herein and to avoid all potential hazards. By following the instructions contained herein, the reader willingly assumes all risks in connection with such instructions.

The Publisher makes no representation or warranties of any kind, including but not limited to, the warranties of fitness for particular purpose or merchantability, nor are any such representations implied with respect to the material set forth herein, and the publisher takes no responsibility with respect to such material. The publisher shall not be liable for any special, consequential, or exemplary damages resulting, in whole or part, from the readers' use of, or reliance upon, this material.

Cover Design: Suzanne McCarron
Cover Photo: James Parker, Parkers Studio

Milady Staff:
Publisher: Catherine Frangie
Acquisitions Editor: Marlene McHugh Pratt
Project Editor: Annette Downs Danaher
Production Manager: Brian Yacur
Production & Art/Design Coordinator: Suzanne McCarron

COPYRIGHT © 1996 Delmar. Milady is an imprint of Delmar, a division of Thomson Learning. Thomson Learning™ is a registered trademark used herein under license.

Printed in the United States of America
8 9 10 11 12 XXX 09 08 07 06 05 04

For more information, contact Milady, 3 Columbia Circle, PO Box 15015, Albany, NY 12212-0515; or find us on the World Wide Web at http://www.Milady.com

ALL RIGHTS RESERVED. No part of this work covered by the copyright hereon may be reproduced or used in any form or by any means—graphic, electronic, or mechanical, including photocopying, recording, taping, Web distribution or information storage and retrieval systems—without the written permission of the publisher.

For permission to use material from this text or product contact us at Tel (800) 730-2214; Fax (800) 730-2215; www.thomsonrights.com

Library of Congress Cataloging-in-Publication Data

Jones, Jamie.
    SalonOvations' braids and updo's made easy / by Jamie Jones.
        p.   cm.
    ISBN 1-56253-318-5
    1. Braids (Hairdressing)   2. Hair-work.   3. Hairstyles.
    1. SalonOvations (Firm)   II. Title.
    TT975.J66   1995
    646.7'245—dc20

TABLE OF CONTENTS

Part 1   The Business of Long Hair Design

Part 2   The Basics of Long Hair Design

Part 3   Working With Long Hair

ACKNOWLEDGMENTS

I would like to express my sincere appreciation for the support, suggestions, and hard work of the following people:

My husband Steven and our children, Jarad and Justin, for their love, devotion and belief in me and my "projects."

Amy O'Brien, for her drawings and her commitment to making the designs easily understood. Her illustrations, patience, honesty, and special attention to detail make this book one I'm proud to put my name on.

James Parker, for the beautiful photographs and his patience in waiting for me to "do it over."

Wendy Webb, for organizing my thoughts, helping to develop and edit the manuscript, and helping me see the difference between speaking and writing.

Leo Passage and Pivot Point International, for constant encouragement and support of my concepts and teaching system. And especially to Leo, a man whose personality, friendship, and dedication to education have greatly affected my life.

Marlene Pratt, for always having or finding out, answers to my many questions about publishing a book. A true professional.

SalonOvations, for believing in my teaching system, and the continued support in sharing those systems through their books and magazines devoted to educating the beauty industry.

Most important, I give thanks for all things unto God.

ABOUT THE AUTHOR

Jamie Rines Jones has been a licensed hairstylist since 1977, with many years of salon experience. She travels extensively teaching long hair design concepts for *Pivot Point International*, as well as her own company, *Helping Hand Productions*.

Founded in 1985, Helping Hand Productions was created with one goal in mind: to produce videotapes and books that take the fear and frustration out of working with long hair. The results of her work are styles completed in 20 minutes or less, without setting and prep work, and minimal to no backcombing. And all of this is done without assistance.

Through on-going workshops, clinics, and show appearances, Jamie has alleviated potential styling problems, and developed special hints for working with long hair. All of the styles have been tested for beauty, simplicity, wearability, and consumer acceptance through her presentations before appearing in a book or video.

Videotapes by Jamie Rines Jones that are currently available include: *Braiding Made Easy, French Braiding Made Easy, Advanced Braiding Made Easy, Ribbon Braiding Made Easy, Updo's Made Easy* and *More Updo's Made Easy.*

PREFACE

How to Use This Book

This book is designed to address long hair styling concerns by answering questions and solving problems quickly and easily. Written for stylists in a salon, as well as those in an academic setting, this book will provide you with the tested and proven answers to the common fears and frustrations that sometimes occur when working with long hair.

Part 1: The Business of Long Hair addresses the need for providing long hair services and the common excuses hairstylists give for avoiding these services. Also, in Part 1, is information on marketing and advertising long hair services.

Part 2: The Basics of Long Hair covers a variety of topics including: shampooing and brushing, tools needed, the use of pins, back-combing, and other essential information.

Part 3: Working With Long Hair covers the step-by-step technical method for creating braids and updo's. Text and illustrations will show you exactly how to achieve a desired style.

Until now there has been no universal format for teaching braids and updo's. The difficulty in mastering these skills have very often been all in the hands. So how do you make your hands do what your eyes see? The answer, very simply, is the *Braiding Made Easy Filing System*: a system Jamie developed that uses the same hand positions throughout a style, or series of styles, and takes the confusion out of working with long hair. *Part 3: Working With Long Hair*, reviews a variety of braids and updo's while using the Filing System to take you through every step in creating beautiful, yet simple, styles.

At the beginning of each technical style section you will find "Jamie's Law," a brief note that corrects common mistakes.

PART 1

The Business of Long Hair

Providing Long Hair Services

Most licensed hairstylists in the United States do not offer long hair services. This presents a problem for the client who calls a full-service salon only to find out the service they want is unavailable. The salon ends up turning this customer away.

In some cases, a salon may have a stylist who offers braids and updo's, but the client calling is yours. Again, since you do not offer the service, the client would be sent to the other stylist.

There are five common excuses hairstylist give when asked why they don't provide long hair services:

1. I never learned how.

2. I tried once but it was so confusing, I couldn't make my hands do what my eyes saw.

3. I don't have long hair clientele.

4. It requires too much time on the salon schedule.

5. I learned once, but never practiced. Now I've forgotten it all.

It can be confusing to learn something new. And sometimes, when we watch someone else work with long hair it seems so simple. Yet when you try it, you suddenly wonder just how many thumbs you really have.

Even though you never learned, or found it too confusing, you have taken the right step in solving this situation. Right now you are reading these pages and starting the process of learning basic and intermediate long hair designs.

To help you in this process, you will find detailed pictures highlighting each strand of hair during each step. Most importantly, you will find that one hand position is used throughout each braid and updo. This takes the difficulty out of manipulating more than one strand of hair.

If you don't have long hair clientele, there are suggestions and solutions available as well. You can find more details on this topic by referring to page 4, "Marketing and Advertising."

The salon schedule issue has been helped by the use of blow drying. As a result, the amount of time a client spends in the salon is greatly reduced. And you'll find that the braids and updo's in this book require no more time in your chair than a blow dry. While there is still a need to do more dressed hair, that is not where you want to begin doing long hair designs.

If you learned how to do braids and updo's, but never practiced, it's time to start. You should practice until you can do the design without thinking about it too much. Consider using a mannequin to practice on between client appointments. When you've perfected the styles, the mannequin is there to display your work. Practice frequently, master the technique, and then you're ready to offer a new service with confidence that each style you do is beautiful every time.

It's hard to get and keep, clients. But by offering total hair care, the reason for sending clients elsewhere is easily removed. Long hair services can be just as easy. Now you can make beautiful braids and long hair designs in twenty minutes or less, without an assistant, setting or prep work, and minimal to no back-combing. And, these styles are wearable for your clients, not *avant-garde* show hair.

With the frustration of working with long hair gone, you can offer total hair care, and keep those clients coming.

Marketing and Advertising

After you have mastered long hair design, now is the time to obtain more long hair clientele. This can be done in a number of ways:

1. Make complimentary service cards.

2. Affiliate yourself with bridal and formal dress shops.

3. Work with bridal and fashion shows.

4. Combine services with special event clothing stores.

5. Create a style photo album.

6. Use mannequins for display.

7. Advertise.

Complimentary service cards are a very effective marketing tool. On the back of your business card write, "One free braid or up-do." Set an expiration date of about two weeks, and add "One coupon per customer." Next, give these cards to women with long hair, and get ready for the phone to ring. When the calls come in for an appointment, ask the client to come in with clean, dry hair. This will save you time.

A simple, easy up-do can be completed in about fifteen minutes. Then, give your client some business cards. Request that when someone asks where she got her hair done, she must give out your card.

This marketing approach can be very effective around prom and homecoming time at your local high school. Give out the complimentary cards with an expiration date one week before the event. This gives your clients the chance to see your work and develop the confidence you can do just what they want. They'll remember you for other special occasions, and tell their friends. This approach is one that guarantees increasing your client list.

Bridal and formal dress shops should not be overlooked. This is a perfect place to put out free service cards and draw new, long hair clients. Let the manager know you'd be interested in doing the hair for any shows she does.

Bridal and fashion shows occur in many cities as a way for models to display the latest fashions. Offer to do all the hair, for free salon advertising. The woman attending these shows will see your talent and could become new clients as well.

Combining services with your salon, formal dress shops, and a tuxedo shop is effective advertising for local high school proms. For example, on a Friday, three weeks before the prom, two male and two female students can be dressed by the tuxedo and dress shops. Hair and make-up can be done by your salon. The students attending school dressed this way will attract a lot of attention, and are more than willing to pass out your business cards. The result is new clients for the salon, including the nail technician, and ultimately many new long-term clients. Retail sales could double and not just through the sale of shampoos and sprays, but through hair accessories that were worked into the final designs.

Photo albums that contain pictures of different long hair designs you've done is another easy, affordable, and very effective way to advertise. The albums, along with your business cards, can be placed in formal dress shops or bridal shops as a way for the long hair client to see your actual work.

Mannequins are perfect for practice and advertising. Put a beautiful style on the mannequin and set it out for the clients to see and talk about. If your client doesn't have long hair, she might have a friend or relative who does.

Advertise your long hair services. You might say something like: "We specialize in long hair," or "We love long hair" in all your printed advertising. Since most salons don't offer long hair services, and you do, don't hesitate to mention this in newspaper ads, flyers and, don't forget, the phone book. This approach will bring in new clients who have never been to your salon before.

Fees for Long Hair Services

Pricing for services is different all over the country. So answering the question of pricing can be difficult.

A general rule of thumb is to charge five dollars above your standard price for long hair services. For example, if you charge fifteen dollars for a shampoo and blowdry, you might want to charge twenty dollars for a shampoo and braid or up-do.

There are times you might not want to charge more for a braid or up-do. For instance, when the client comes in with clean, dry hair and your design takes only takes 15 minutes, a lesser fee might be more acceptable. Or, if a client is on the book for a shampoo, cut and blowdry, and you suggest a shampoo, cut and braid instead, then you may not want to charge extra for this.

But, most importantly, keep in mind what your market will bear:

1. In order to charge more for long hair services, you want to offer clients something they can't do by themselves.

2. There are some cases where a client is not able to pay for extra services, yet could be great advertisement with a braid.

3. There are some situations where a client will gladly pay to have a look different from anyone else.

These are important considerations when determining pricing for this type of service. Keep them in mind when deciding what is best for you and your client.

PART 2

The Basics of Long Hair

Shampooing and Brushing

Shampooing and brushing long hair requires special techiques that not only make it easier for you but also causes less damage to long hair.

It is best for long hair to be shampooed in a standing position. This reduces tangling. So if a client's hair is shampooed at home before she arrives at your salon, it saves you both time. Therefore, it is suggested that a client use products recommended by you that are best for her, and that she arrives at the salon with clean, dry hair.

If your client requires a shampoo, use a gentle, all hair-type shampoo. With damaged or chemically treated hair, a moisturizing shampoo should be used, followed by a weekly, deep penetrating conditioner. There are several products available from professional haircare companies, and the choice is a matter of personal preference.

When laying your client back in the shampoo bowl, place the hair into the bowl with the least amount of tangling possible. Wet the hair on the scalp first and then let the water run to the ends. Apply shampoo to the scalp only, then massage the entire scalp area using small circular motions. Now, rinse the hair while working the shampoo through to the ends. This is usually all that's required to cleanse the ends, since the primary goal is to clean the scalp without tangling the ends of the hair. Following this shampooing technique will cut down on the time needed for detangling and combing the hair.

Sit your client up, and towel blot the hair by placing the towel over sections of the hair. Start at the top and squeeze as you work your way down. Do not rub. Rubbing will not remove excess water, but will instead create matting of the ends.

Change the towel whenever it gets too wet. Expect to use several towels.

At this point a leave-in conditioner is strongly recommended. Use of this product will make combing the hair much easier. It also helps hold moisture in the hair when exposed to the heat of the sun, or the cold drying weather of winter.

To comb long hair, start at the ends and gently work out the tangles while moving up one inch at a time. A large toothed, bone comb is effective to detangle the hair when it is wet. If the client comes in with clean, dry hair, a large paddle brush works well. Use the same technique of starting at the bottom and working up in one-inch increments.

Now it's time to dry the hair. Usually a blowdryer is used while running your fingers through the hair from the scalp to the ends. Always go in the direction of the cuticle layer not against it. If you need to save some time, put your client under a hairdryer for about five minutes to remove excess water.

Wet or Dry?

If possible, it is best to work with dry hair. The only exception would be one where the client wanted a style that wasn't the best for her hair type. In this case, the hair requires dampening with water in a spray bottle, and adding gel or mousse, to hold the hair in place.

Working with dry hair means the client doesn't have to walk around with wet hair. Also, as hair dries, it shrinks. If a braid is comfortable while the hair is wet, it will get tighter and uncomfortable as the hair dries. This could cause a headache for the client, which might result in your loss of a customer.

Some stylists like to work with wet, gelled hair because it is easier to make it neat. This is true only if you have not perfected a hand position that stops the hair from sliding as you work with it. This hand technique will be discussed further in the book, and you will find that wet hair is no longer required to achieve neatness.

Tools of the Trade

There are only two tools needed to work with long hair. They are:

1. A large 11" tail comb.

2. A square paddle brush.

The large tail comb is eleven inches long, and is made of bone with 1/4" of space between the teeth. It is used for detangling wet hair and for back-combing dry hair. The tail portion of this comb is 6" long, which is required for making entire head sections. It is also long enough to hold all the hair at one time.

The square, anti-static, paddle brush is perfect for long hair for three reasons: First, these brushes usually have flexible rubber bristles. If you are brushing the hair and come to a knot, the tip will bend and release the hair rather than ripping through the knot which causes breakage. Second, the rubber bristles are seated in a padded base which gives when pressure is applied. This adds to the assurance that the hair is not damaged or broken. And finally, removing hair from these brushes is easier than with other brushes.

These are the only tools necessary when creating the long hair designs you'll find in this book. If you find other tools that work better for you, feel free to use them.

Back-combing

Teasing with great vigor was taught in school at one time. It was achieved by using a teasing brush and brushing hard against the cuticle layer from the scalp to the ends. It resulted in very matted, tangled hair. This is not necessary with the styles you will be doing in this book. These styles use no teasing, but a few will require small amounts of back-combing.

Back-combing is done by placing a comb underneath a strand of hair. Starting very close to the base, roll the comb and apply medium pressure going against the cuticle layer. Usually back-combing a strand once or twice is all that is needed to create the fullness required for these styles. Your goal is to make the strand you are back-combing fuller, and to prevent it from splitting or opening when you work with that strand.

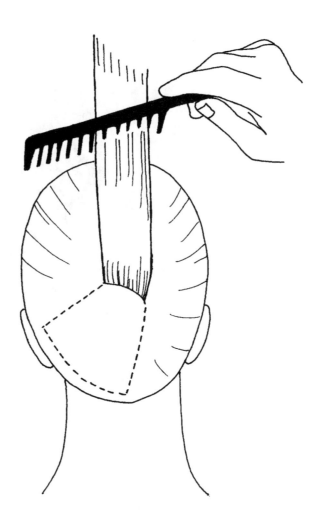

Remember, *back-combing should always be done with the hair combed in the direction you want the hair to go when finished.* Here is a common mistake seen in back-combing:

Say the hair is in a ponytail at the crown, and you want to place a curl behind the left ear. The stylist very often will back-comb the hair straight up, then try to force it behind the left ear. The result is usually buckling, or unevenness of that hair strand.

Now, taking this same example with proper back-combing:

Section out the hair you want placed behind the left ear, then comb it in the direction you want the hair to lay. Next, back-comb this strand while keeping it in this position. Place your comb underneath and starting very close to the base, back-comb the strand by rolling the comb while applying medium pressure. Smooth out the top if necessary then place the strand where you want it. If you are making a curl, there is no need to back-comb the ends since they will be tucked under.

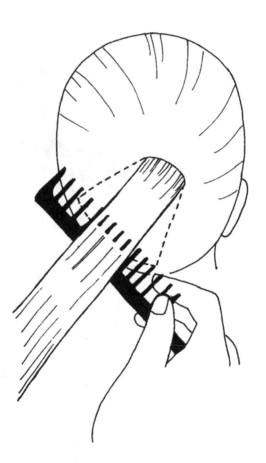

Bobby Pins vs Hairpins

Bobby pins and hairpins look similar yet have a completely different purpose.

Bobby pins touch in the middle, and are designed to hold weight. They are best suited when you need to anchor a weighted curl, or when you change the direction of the hair such as in the Bowtie (page 144) or the French Twist with backcombing (page 151). For direction changes, make sure the tips cross each other. This gives them added strength in holding the hair where you want it.

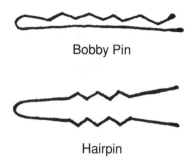

Bobby Pin

Hairpin

Hairpins are used to help place hair that has already been secured with a bobby pin. For example, once a curl has been placed and secured where you want it, you might decide to spread the curl to make it wider. Spread the hair with your fingers, then secure with a hairpin to hold the strands in the new position.

A common question concerns the placement of pins in the hair. A basic rule is to pin exactly where your fingers are holding the hair. Very often bobby pins are being inserted next to the fingers holding the hair. When the stylist lets go, the hair moves to the new pinned position. It takes a little practice, but it's worth it for perfect style placement everytime.

The styles that follow in this book, will offer examples for the use of bobby pins and hairpins. Suggestions will be made for the best pin to use.

The Perfect Ponytail

One of the most common problems stylists run into is getting the ponytail exactly where they want it while keeping the hair smooth. The main reason the hair doesn't stay smooth is because stylists try to tighten it after rubber band placement. Following are two different ways to make a ponytail without ever tightening it. Try both, then decide which works best for you.

PONYTAIL #1
You will need 2 bobby pins and an elastic band (preferably fabric covered).

1. Attach two bobby pins to rubberband as shown.

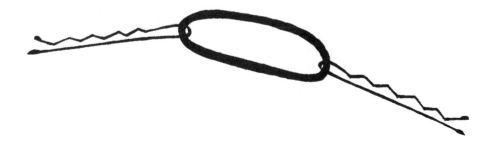

2. Put left hand where you want ponytail to be placed and brush hair into it. Holding hair securely, twist ponytail 1/4 turn clockwise.

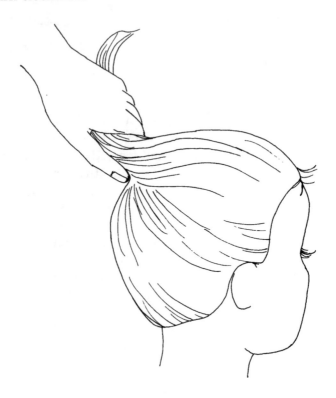

3. Insert one bobby pin into the top of the ponytail next to scalp. Hold securely with index finger. Allow other bobby pin to hang freely on the right side of ponytail.

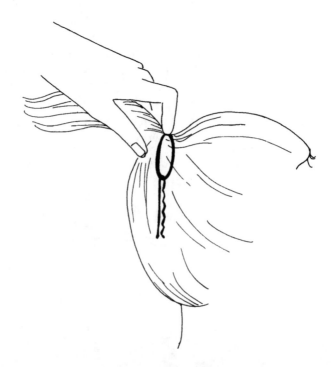

4. With right arm, reach over top of ponytail. With right hand, reach under ponytail to grab free hanging bobby pin. Pull rubberband at least 1-1/2 times around ponytail.

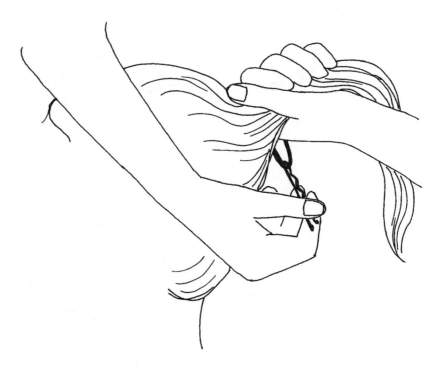

5. Insert free bobby pin into ponytail under the rubberband along the scalp.

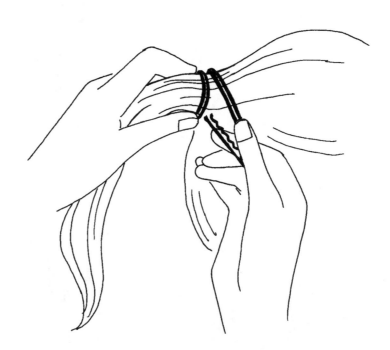

PONYTAIL #2
You will need 1 bobby pin and 1 rubberband (preferably fabric covered).

1. Attach bobby pin to rubberband as shown.

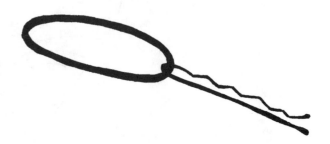

2. Put your left hand where you want the ponytail to be placed and brush hair into it. Hook the rubberband over your left thumb and allow the bobby pin to hang free.

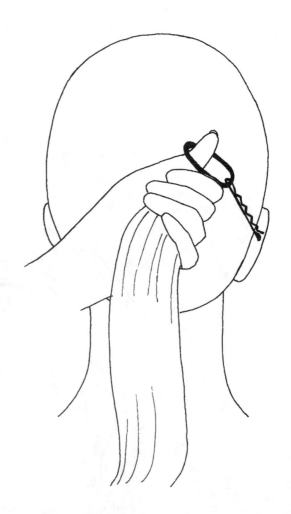

3. With your right hand, grab the free-hanging bobby pin and pull it underneath the ponytail, then pull bobby pin through the rubberband.

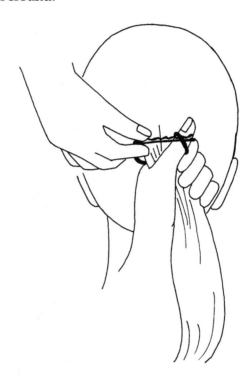

4. Pull the bobby pin back underneath the ponytail, and go back around the ponytail at least one time.

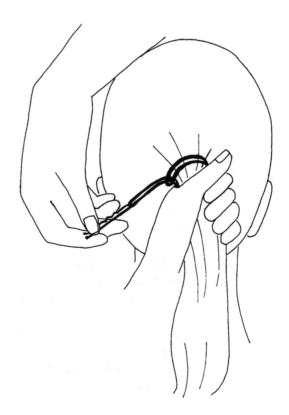

5. Insert free bobby pin into ponytail between the rubberband and scalp.

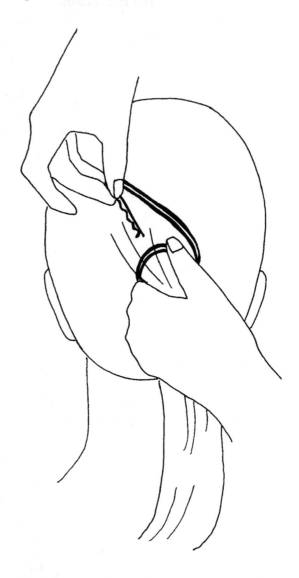

Accessories

Some of the following styles use ribbon to create the finished look. Here are some questions commonly asked about purchasing ribbon.

How wide should the ribbon be? The styles in this book use a ribbon no wider that 1/2". A personal favorite is 1/4" wide. It is easier to work with and it doesn't make the style quite as stiff.

What kind of ribbon is best? The ribbon should be as slick as possible. Metallic ribbons are fun, but they rarely have a smooth finish. When the ribbon is not smooth, it can pull on the hair and make the style look messy. The perfect test for ribbon is to run it over a silky fabric or panty hose and see if it catches. Once you have perfected using ribbons, you can successfully use ribbons that are not as slick, and still keep the style clean.

How long should the ribbon be? It is best to start with ribbon at least twice the length of hair you are working on. Many of the styles don't require quite that much, but nothing could be worse than getting to the end of a style and finding out you need just a couple inches more. Better safe than sorry, so cut the ribbon twice the hair length to be sure.

Is there anything else besides ribbon that can be used? Yes, strings of pearls and strings of sequins can be used successfully. You can purchase these at most fabric or craft stores. They come on spools of five yards or more and can be cut to any length. But, again, you will not want to work with these two accessories until you have mastered using smooth ribbon. You will have a much better chance of a successful design.

You should always keep extra ribbon in your salon. There may be times a client comes in for a long hair design and has not thought of a hair accessory. By having a few extra yards of black, white, gold and silver you will be prepared.

While you are at the fabric or craft center, take time to look around. There are always treasures to be found and used in your salon. Some highly recommended items include:

Individual beads and pearls. These are easily put onto a hairpin and placed in the finished design to dress it up. Colors recommended are gold, black, silver, and opaque white. Sizes recommended are from 2 to 4mm. Following are directions for putting beads on hairpins and using them in your long hair designs.

1. Straighten a hairpin and slide bead onto it.

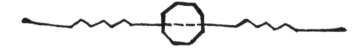

2. Bend the hairpin down firmly on either side of bead.

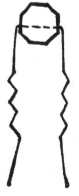

3. Bend one leg of the hairpin halfway up, as shown. This prevents the hairpin from slipping out when worn. Slide this accessorized pin into any hairstyle that needs to be dressed up for a special occasion.

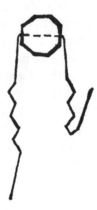

4. You can also tie bows or ribbons on the hairpin for a different look.

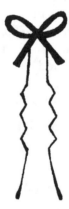

Easier still is to buy them already tied and just slip them onto a pin.

Silk flowers You can purchase tiny flowers wrapped in a small bundle. These are great to have on hand. In the salon just cut them out of the bundle and insert into the final design. If you use hairspray after you insert the flowers it will help hold them in place. Real flowers, like baby's breath, are wonderful too, but these are difficult to have on hand all the time.

Buttons Some of the buttons available today are tiny works of art. You can always hot glue or sew these onto a fabric-covered rubberband for a dressy or more fun look. Small rhinestone buttons can be added to a hairpin (follow directions for individual beads and pearls) for a stunning finish to an evening design.

Once you start looking around you will become creative and come up with your own ideas. Belt buckles, tee-shirt clasps and even gold charms have been used before, so don't be limited by the few things mentioned here.

Always have ready-made hair accessories available. These provide good retail sales year around. Many clients who were not even thinking of a hair accessory could see something that catches their eye and buy it on impulse. Try to incorporate one in each long hair design that leaves the salon.

PART 3

Working
with
Long Hair

How to Use Part 3

Part 3 is designed to take you through a series of styles. The best way to use Part 3 is as follows:

1. *Start at the beginning.*

   Part 3 of this book is designed so that you master one style before you proceed to the next. Each additional step is based on some technique learned in the style before it.

2. *Copy hand positions exactly.*

   This is the most difficult part in learning how to manipulate two or more sections of hair at one time. Illustrations appear at every step to help you master the hand positions and technique of every style.

3. *Practice, practice, practice.*

   Don't give up if it gets confusing. Start at step #1 again, and make your hands match the illustrations exactly. Keep practicing until the hand positions become comfortable before you move to the next style.

4. *Jamie's Law.*

   Before you start the steps for each style, you will see a special note called, "Jamie's Law." Jamie's Law addresses the most common mistakes made when doing that particular style. If you run into problems, or the style doesn't look right, go back and read Jamie's Law and you will probably find information on the problem area.

STYLE 1

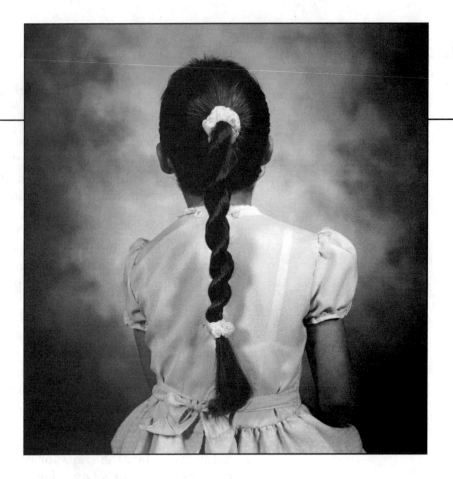

Rope Ponytail and Chignon

The Rope Ponytail is a true show stopper. The concept is simple, yet figuring out how to stop two twisted strands from coming unwound can be difficult. In order for two strands to stay twisted they must go in opposing directions. Notice the left hand side is twisted to the right yet the entire ponytail is twisted to the left.

This braid is best done on all one-length hair.

Jamie's Law: The most common mistake made with this technique is twisting the left-hand side of the ponytail counter clockwise (or to the left). This will result in the twist unwinding. If this happens start over and make sure you twist the left-hand side of the ponytail clockwise (or to the right).

1. Begin with hair in ponytail. Divide ponytail in two sections.

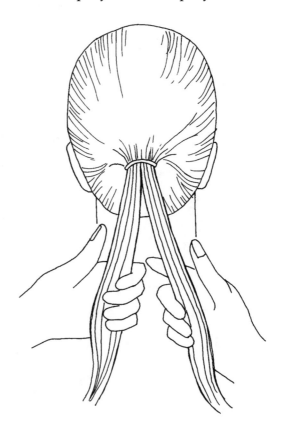

2. Twist left strand clockwise (to the right) two or three times.

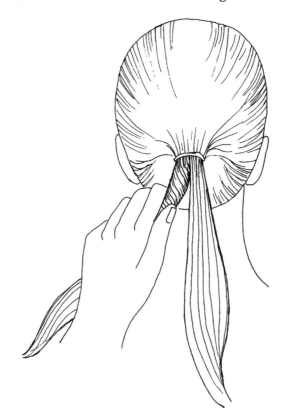

3. Place section in your right hand with index finger inbetween, palm up, as shown.

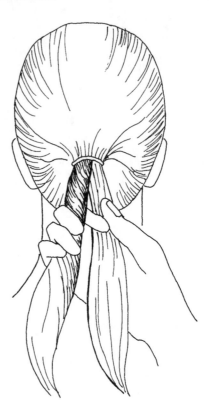

4. Twist palm down (counterclockwise) right strand over left.

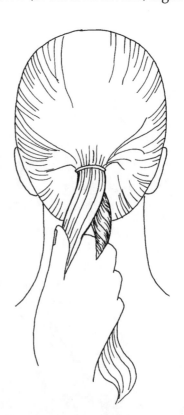

5. Repeat steps 2 through 4 until the ponytail is completely twisted. When this technique is done correctly, you can put a rubberband around the end and it will not come unwound.

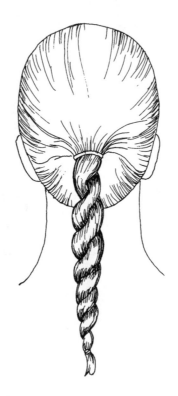

6. Another option is to make a chignon from this rope. Begin twisting the rope ponytail counterclockwise around the rubberband.

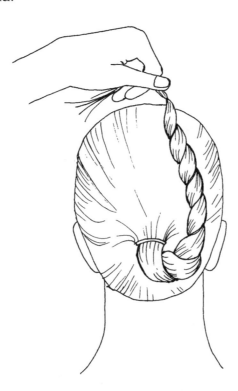

7. When you finish wrapping into a chignon, tuck ends under and secure with bobbypins.

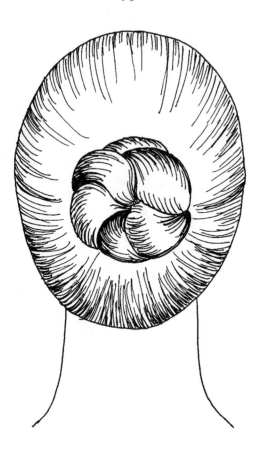

STYLE 2

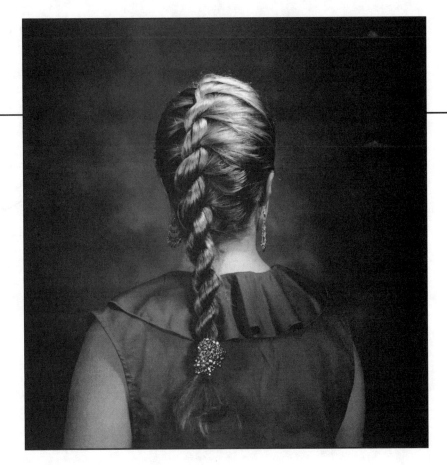

Rope Braid

The rope braid is one most requested for demonstration during workshops and clinics. It can be done on all one-length hair as well as long, layered hair.

Jamie's Law: You must add to both sides before you twist the right side over the left.

1. Take a triangle section of hair from the front. If there are bangs, begin behind them.

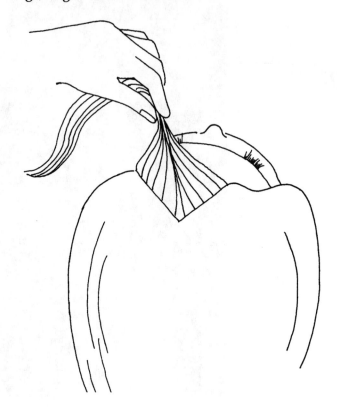

2. Divide the section into two strands.

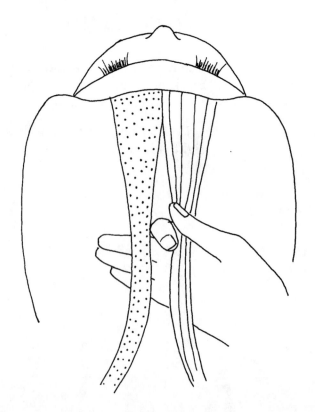

3. Cross the right strand over the left strand.

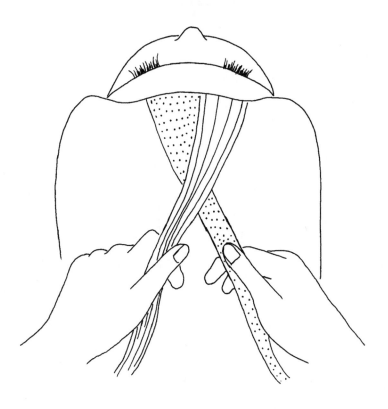

4. Place both strands in the right hand with the index finger inbetween, palm up, as shown.

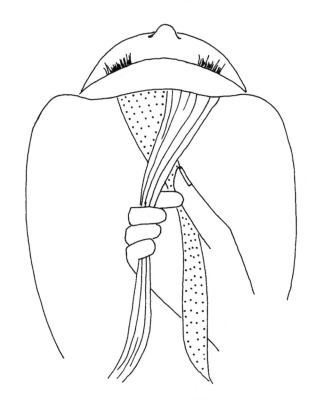

5. Twist the left strand two times clockwise or toward the center.

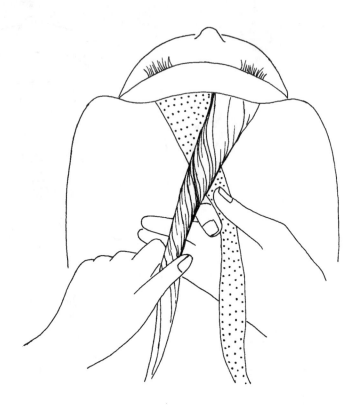

6. Pick up a 1" section from the left side.

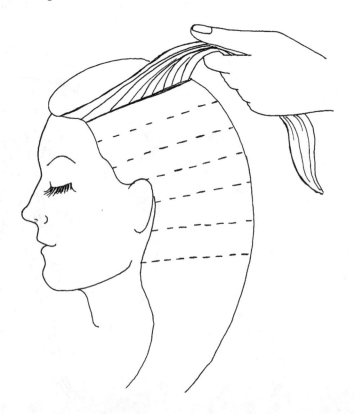

7. Add this section to the left strand.

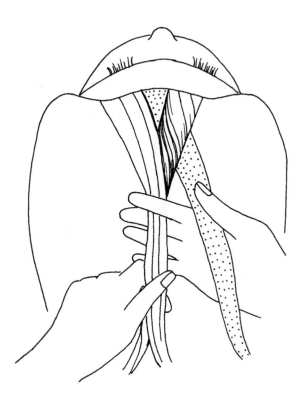

8. Put both strands in the left hand with the index finger inbetween, palm up, as shown.

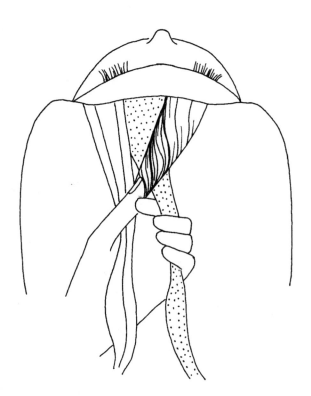

9. Pick up a 1" section from the right side.

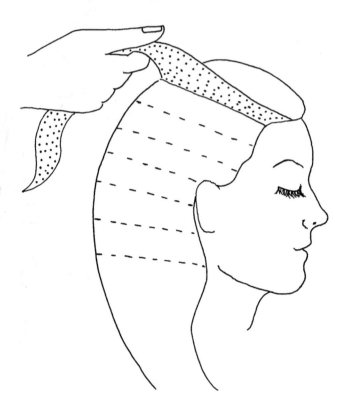

10. Add this section to the right side.

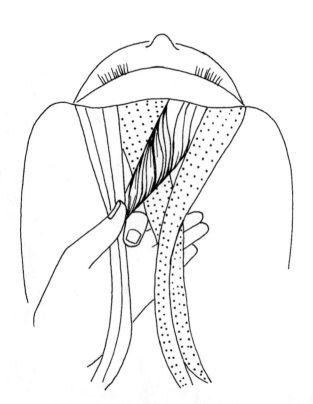

11. Put both strand in the right hand with the index finger in-between, palm up, as shown.

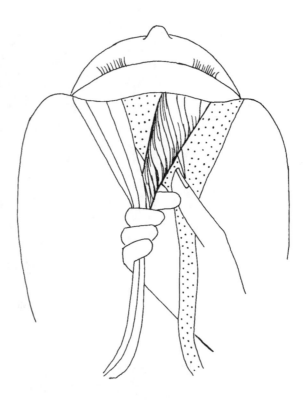

12. With your hand in this position, twist toward the left (counterclockwise) until your palm is facing down.

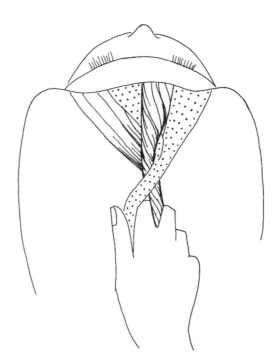

13. Repeat steps 4 through 11 working toward the nape until style is done. Use a rubberband to secure.

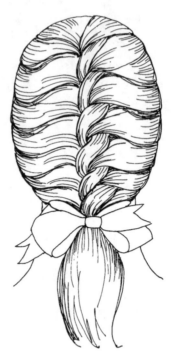

14. When you run out of sections to pick up, you can repeat steps 2 through 4 of the rope ponytail (see page 26). This will lock the braid from coming unwound. Place a rubberband around the ends and let the ponytail hang free.

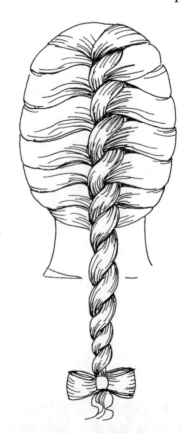

15. Another option would be to bobby pin the ends under in the nape area.

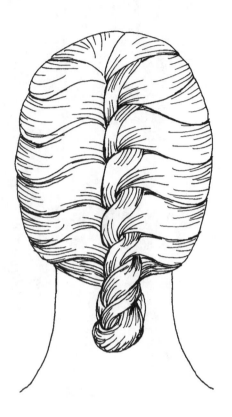

STYLE 3

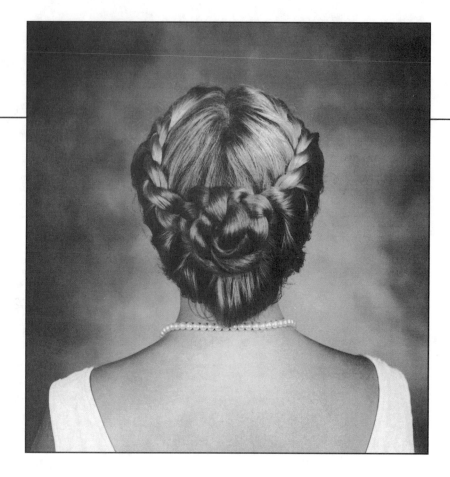

2-Strand Twist

The 2-strand twist is one of the most popular braids. It allows fullness on the sides and behind the ear, and is perfect for the non-oval face. This style is done best on all one-length hair, or shoulder length and longer.

Jamie's Law: You must twist up toward the part. On the right side of the head the right hand does the twisting toward the part and on the left side, the left hand does the work.

1. Divide hair in two sections.

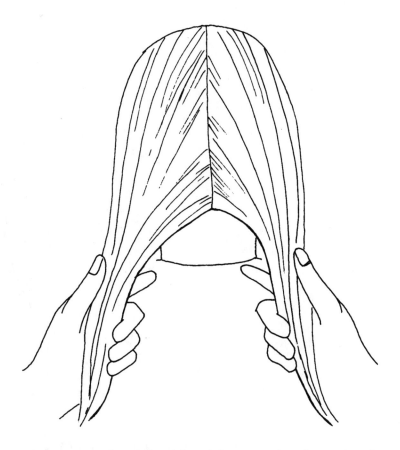

2. Starting on the right side, pick up a triangle section from the front.

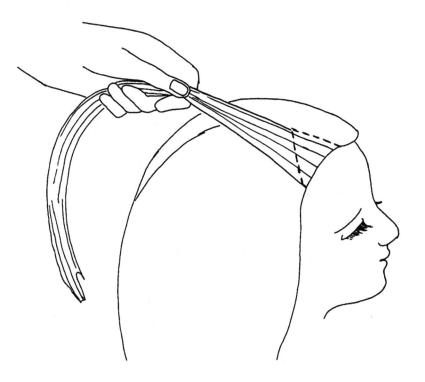

3. Divide this section in two strands.

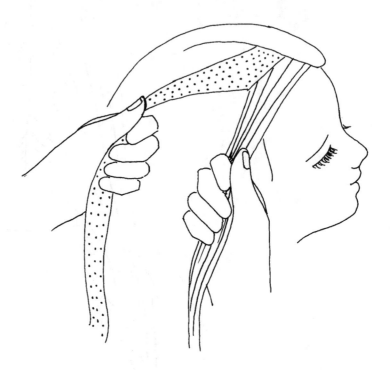

4. Cross the right strand over the left.

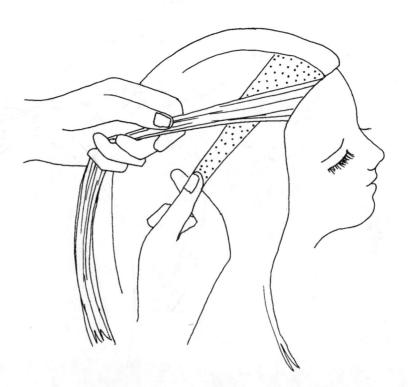

5. Place both strands in the left hand with the index finger inbetween. Keep the back of the left hand against the head at all times.

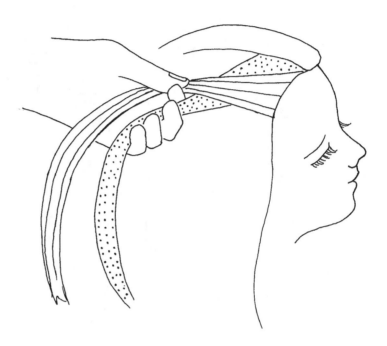

6. Starting at the hairline and continuing up toward your left hand, pick up a 1" section with your right hand.

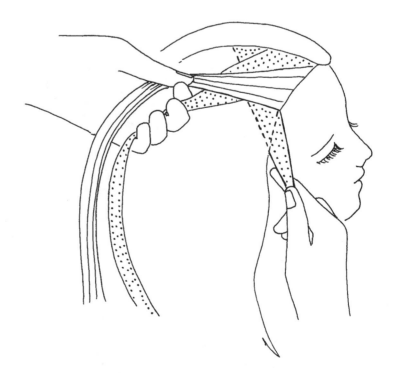

7. Add this section to the right (or bottom) strand.

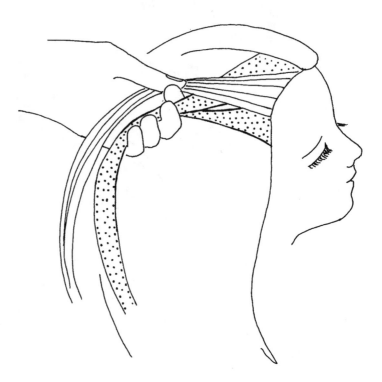

8. Place these sections in your right hand, with the index finger inbetween.

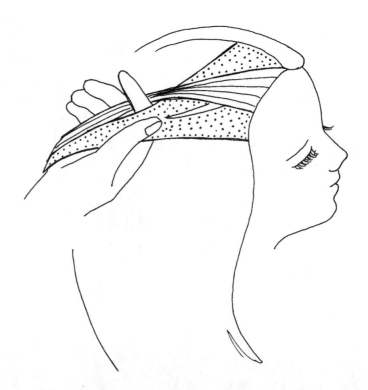

9. Twist right hand counterclockwise (the right strand twists over the left strand).

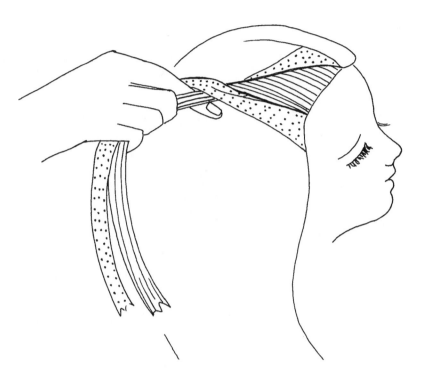

10. Repeat steps 5 through 9, picking up 1" sections of hair as you move down the head. Continue until you reach the nape and have no more hair to pick up. Clip this section out of your way.

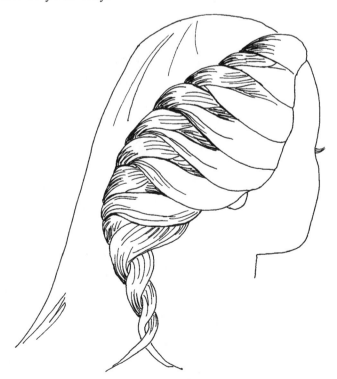

11. Starting on the left side, pick up a triangular section from the front.

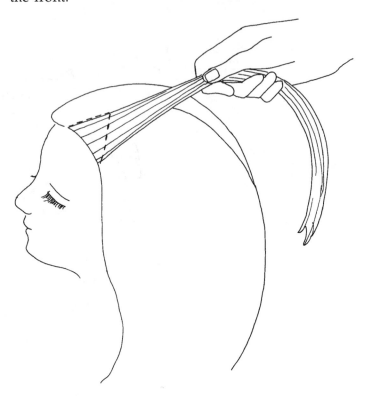

12. Divide this section in two strands.

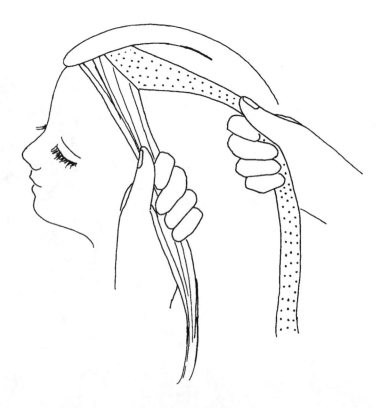

13. Cross the left strand over the right.

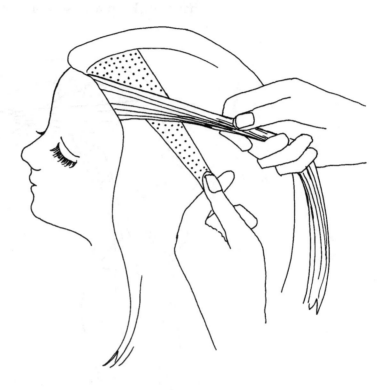

14. Place both strands in the right hand with the index finger inbetween. Keep the back of the right hand against the head at all times.

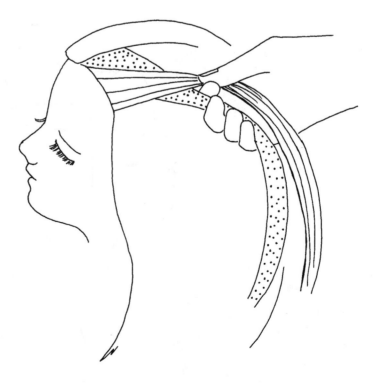

15. Starting at the hairline and continuing up toward your right hand, pick up a 1" section with your left hand.

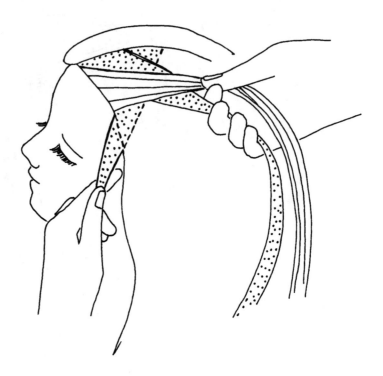

16. Add this section to the left (or bottom) strand.

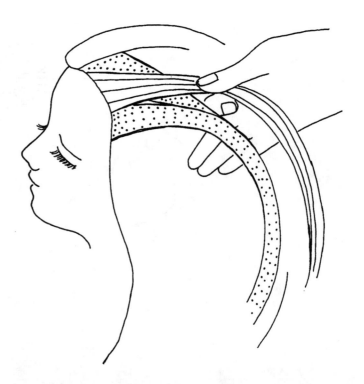

17. Place these sections in your left hand, index finger in-between.

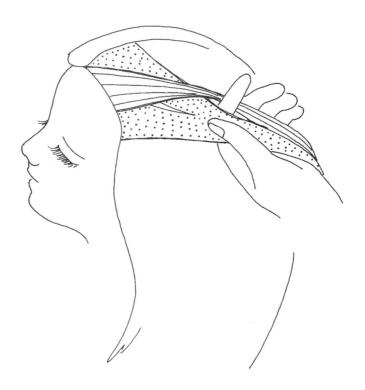

18. Twist left hand clockwise (the left strand twists over the right strand).

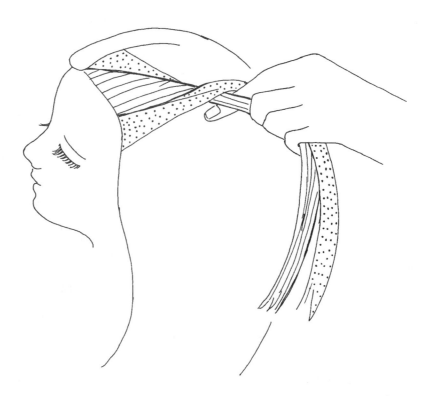

19. Repeat steps 14 through 18, picking up 1" sections of hair as you move down the head. Continue until you reach the nape and run out of hair. Bring both finished sides together to form a ponytail. Secure with a rubberband.

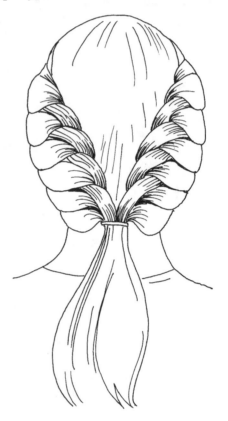

20. Another option would be to do the Fishtail Ponytail. Cover the rubberband with hair, make the ponytail and then pin ends underneath. See style 6 for more information.

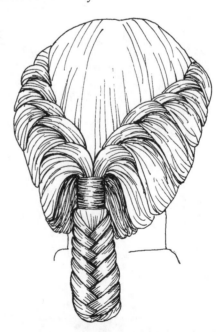

21. You could also leave the back down and do the 2-strand twist on the top portion of the head. This is a great option for all one-length, bob-line haircuts.

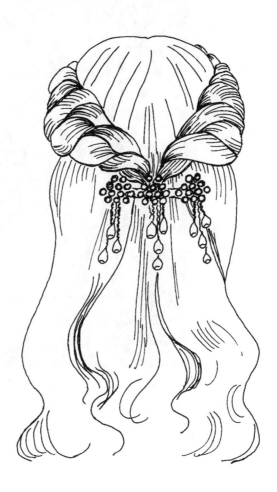

STYLE 4

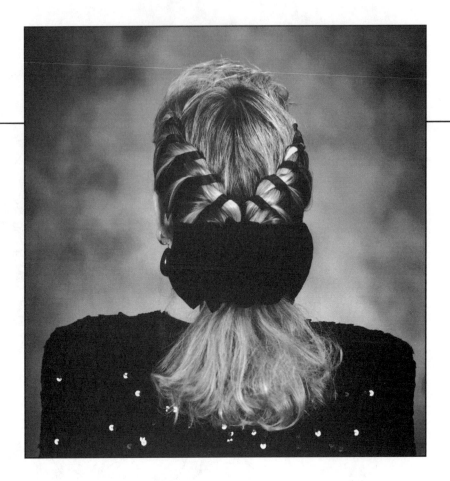

2-Strand Twist with Ribbon

This is another beautiful way to dress up the 2-strand twist. Make sure you have perfected the 2-strand twist without ribbon before you attempt this version. It makes it so much easier to master.

Jamie's Law: The ribbon never gets added to the hair strands. It is always passed *after* you twist the two hair strands over each other and before you pick up your next section.

1. Divide hair in two section as shown.

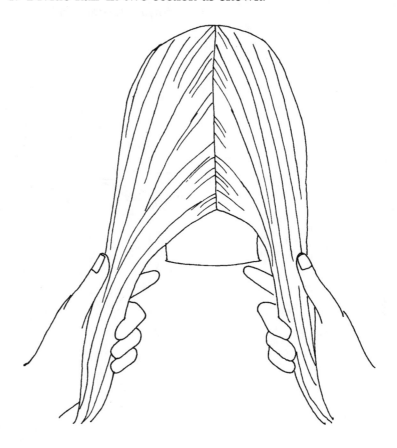

2. Starting on the right side, pick up a triangle section from the front.

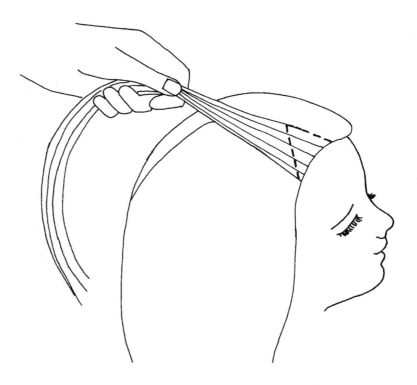

3. Tie a ribbon to the inside of the triangle section. Push the ribbon toward the face and out of the way of the hair sections.

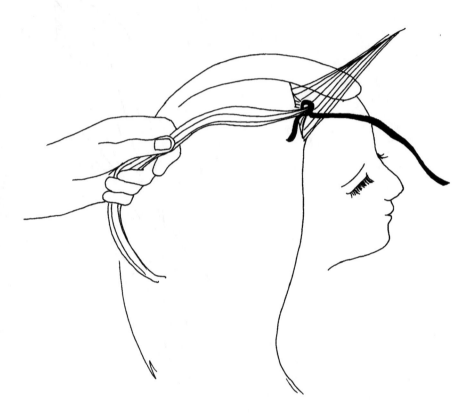

4. Divide the hair section into two strands.

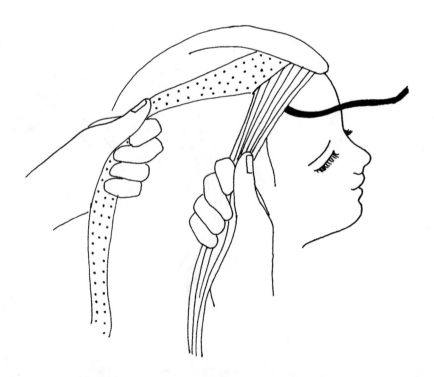

5. Cross the right strand over the left.

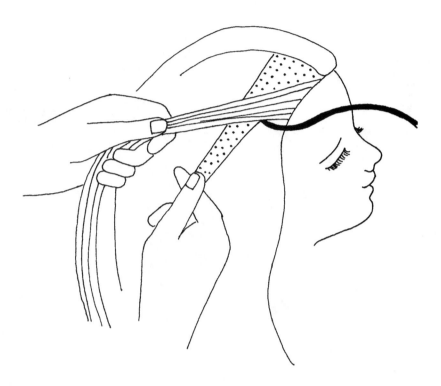

6. Place both strands in the left hand with the index finger inbetween. Keep the back of the left hand against the head at all times.

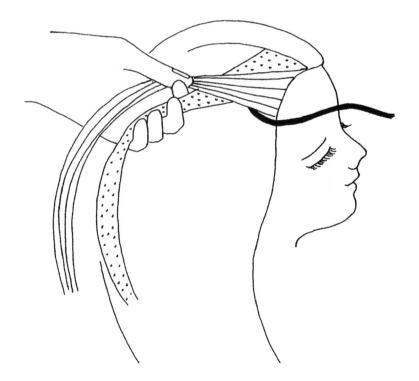

7. Now wrap ribbon counterclockwise completely around both sections. Push ribbon toward the face and out of the way of the hair section.

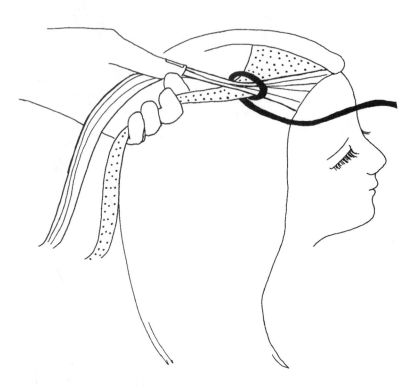

8. Starting at the hairline and continuing up toward your left hand; pick up a 1" section with your right hand.

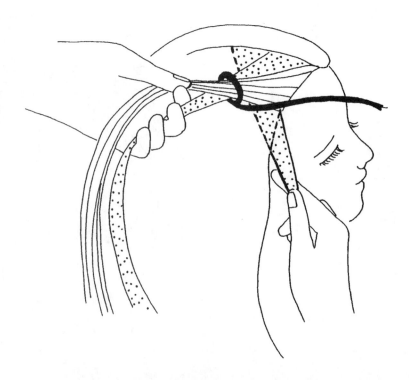

9. Add this section to the right (or bottom) strand.

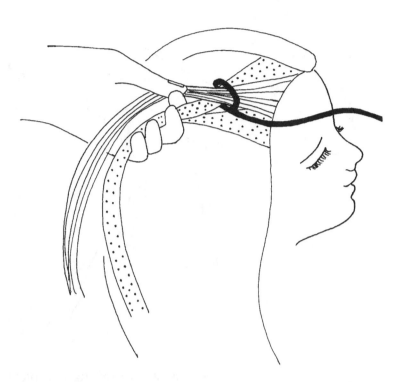

10. Place these sections in your right hand, with the index finger inbetween.

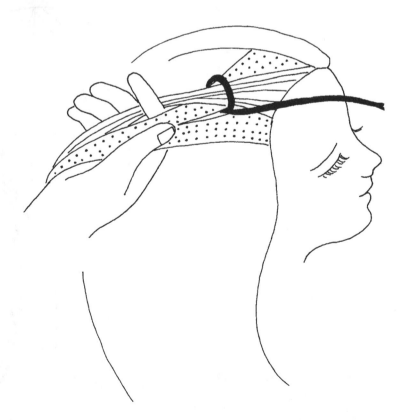

11. Twist right hand counterclockwise (the right strand twists over the left strand).

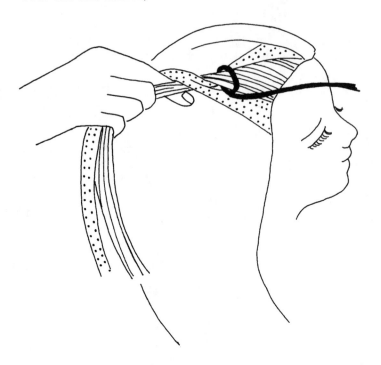

12. Repeat steps 6 through 11, picking up 1" sections of hair as you move down the head. Continue until you reach the nape and have no more hair to pick up.

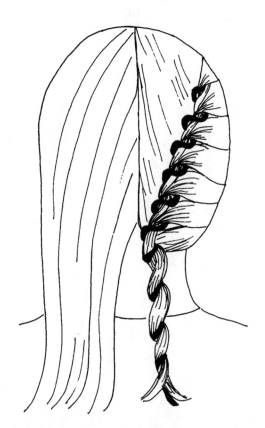

13. Starting on the left side, pick up a triangular section from the front.

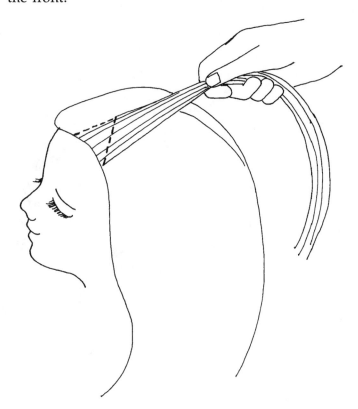

14. Tie a ribbon to the inside of the triangle section. Push ribbon toward the face and out of the way of the hair sections.

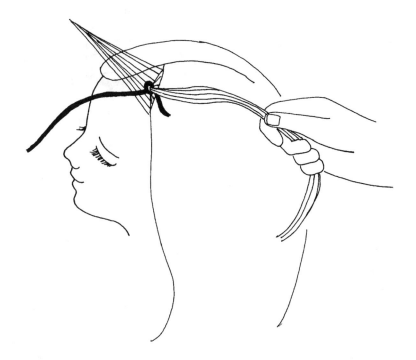

15. Divide the triangle section into two strands.

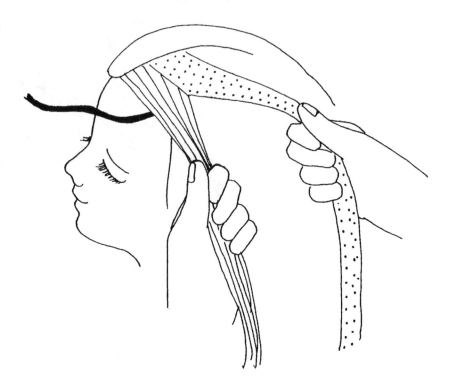

16. Cross the left strand over the right.

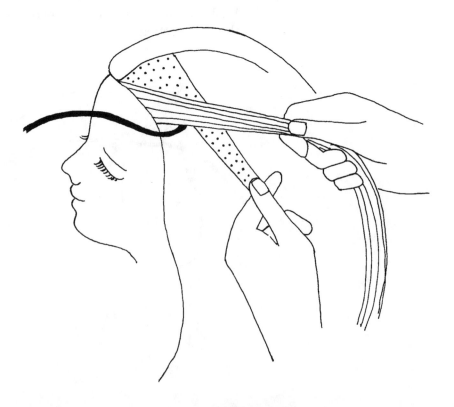

17. Place both strands in the right hand with the index finger inbetween. Keep the back of the right hand against the head at all times.

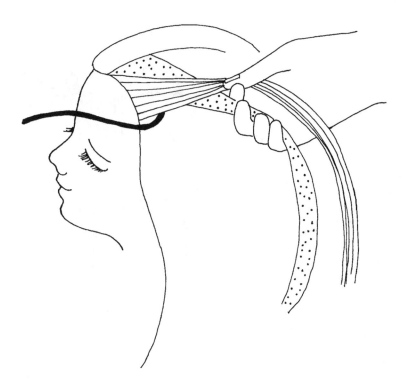

18. Wrap ribbon clockwise completely around both sections. Push ribbon forward and out of the way of the hair strands.

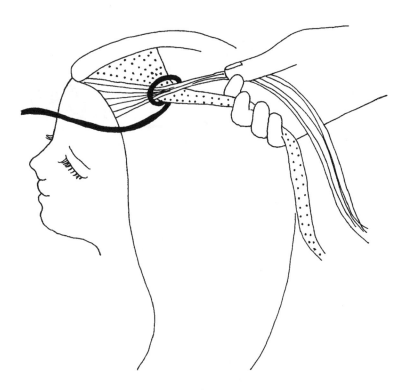

19. Starting at the hairline and continuing up toward your right hand, pick up a 1" section with your left hand.

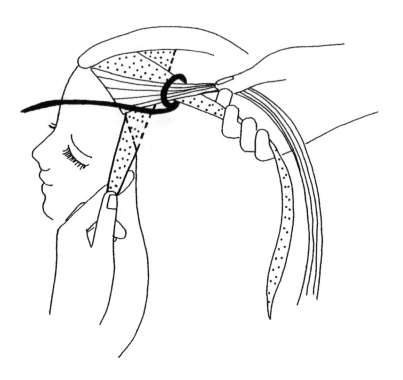

20. Add this section to the left (or bottom) strand.

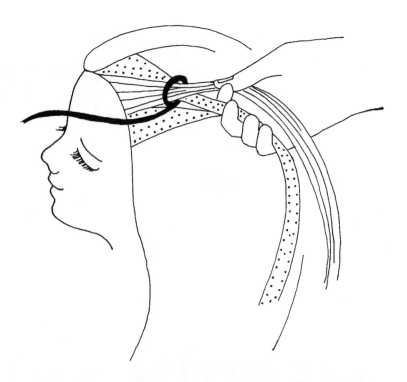

21. Place these sections in your left hand, index finger in-between.

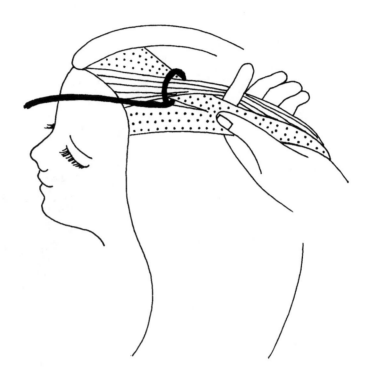

22. Twist left hand clockwise; left strand twists over the right strand).

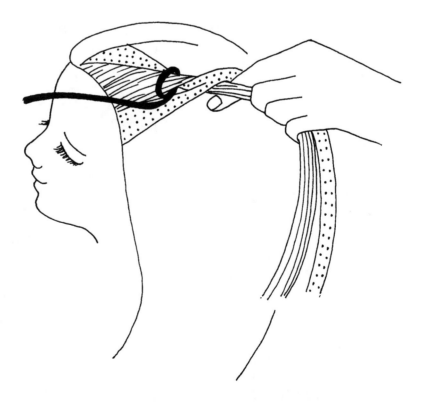

23. Repeat steps 17 through 22, picking up 1" sections of hair as you move down the head. Continue until you reach the nape and run out of hair. Bring both finished sides together to form a ponytail.

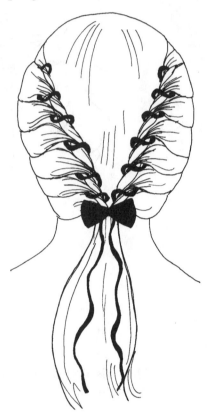

24. Another option would be to wrap both ponytail sections with remaining ribbon, then wrap into a chignon.

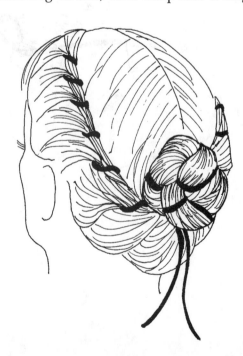

STYLE 5

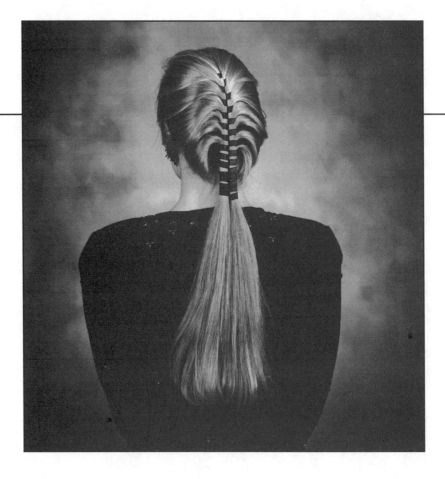

2-Strand Ribbon Braid

This is a perfect style for all one-length hair. It is popular for proms and weddings because ribbon can be braided into the hair to match the dress. It is also very easy to do.

Jamie's Law: The hair strands *never* twist or cross each other. The ribbon does all the work by making a figure 8 around the two strands.

1. Take a triangle section of hair from the front. If there are bangs, begin behind them.

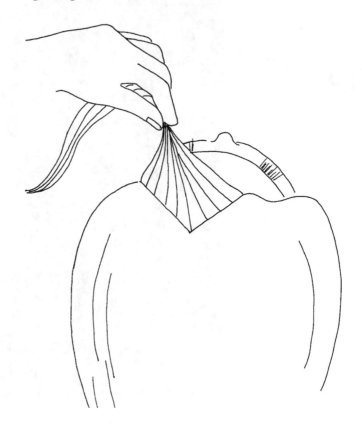

2. Divide the section into two strands. Tie a ribbon onto the left side strand.

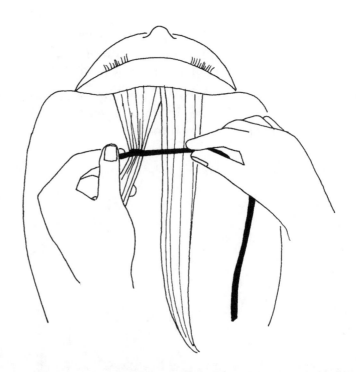

3. While holding the left hand strand, drop the ribbon down to hang freely.

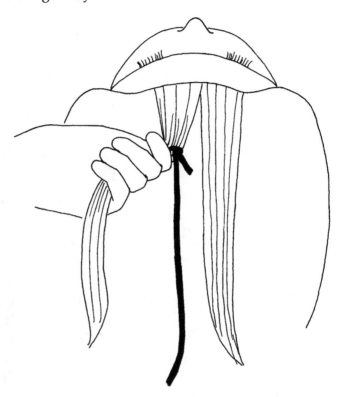

4. Pick up the right strand and place it inbetween the index and third fingers, palm up, as shown. Pick up the ribbon with your right hand and bring it under the right strand.

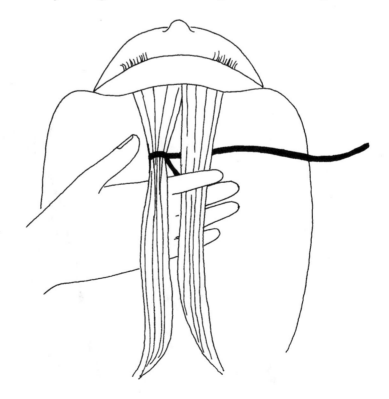

5. Then bring ribbon up and over the right strand. Drop the ribbon to hang freely between the two strands.

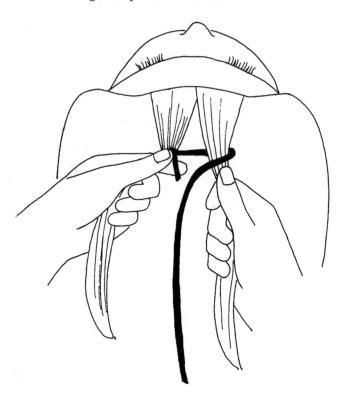

6. Place both strands in your right hand, index finger in-between, palm up, as shown. Allow ribbon to hang freely.

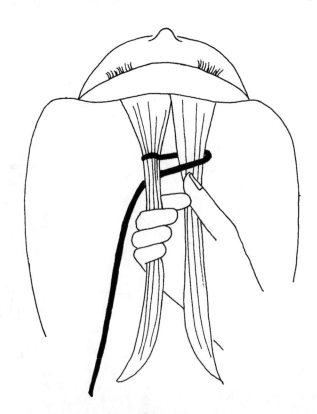

7. Pick up a 1" section on the left side.

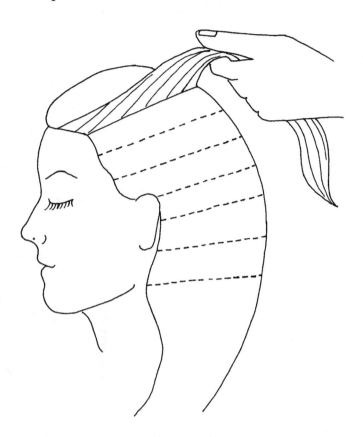

8. Add this section to the left strand you already have in your hand.

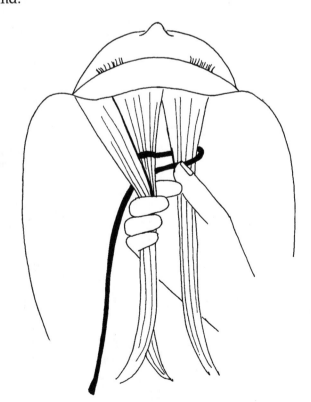

9. Pick up the ribbon with your left hand and bring it under the left strand.

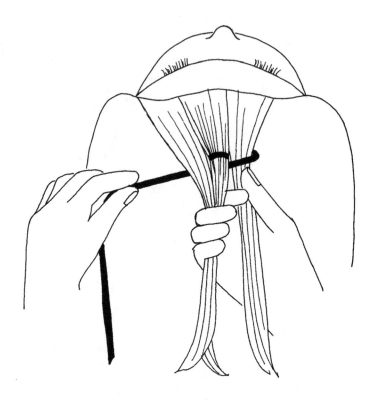

10. Then bring ribbon up and over the left strand. Drop the ribbon to hang freely between the two strands.

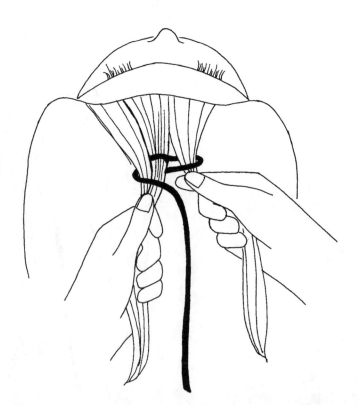

11. Place both strands in your left hand, index finger inbetween, palm up, as shown. Allow ribbon to hang free.

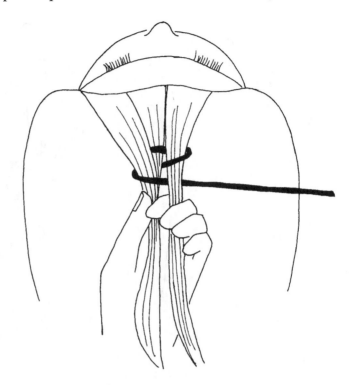

12. Pick up a 1" section on the right side.

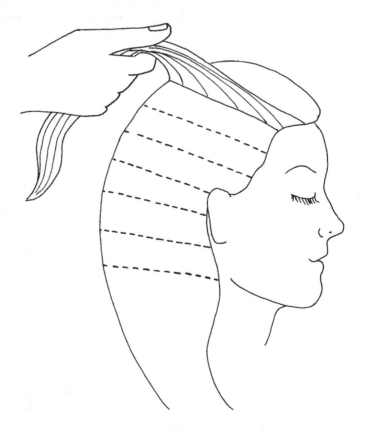

13. Add the section to the right side strand already in your hand.

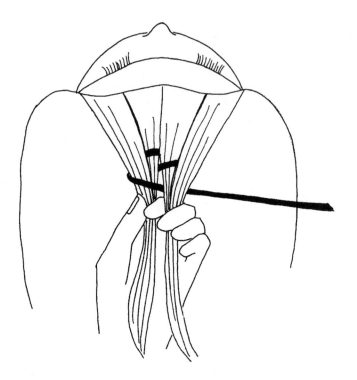

14. Pick up the ribbon with your right hand and bring it under then up and over the right strand. Allow ribbon to hang freely between the two strands.

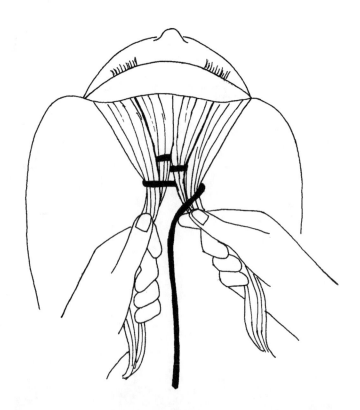

15. Repeat steps 6 through 14 moving down toward the nape with each 1" section picked up. When you run out of sections, secure with rubberband. Remainder of hair forms a ponytail.

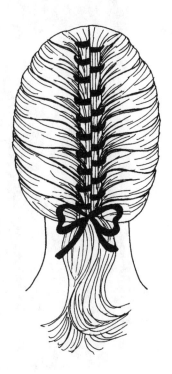

16. Or finish the ponytail by continuing to make a figure 8 with the ribbon to the ends of the hair.

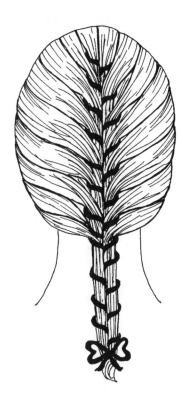

STYLE 6

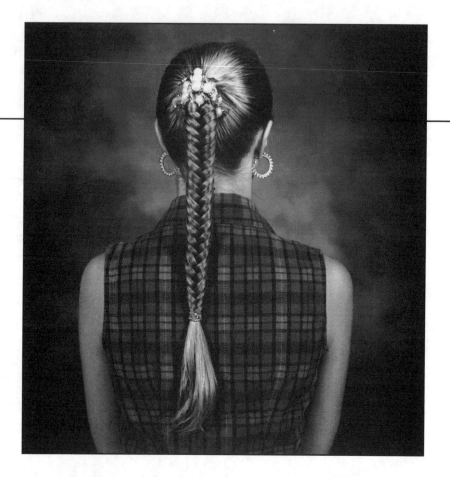

Fishtail Ponytail

The Fishtail is a very complicated looking braid yet is actually one of the easiest braids to do. It is best done on dry, all one-length hair. It makes a very attractive ponytail by itself. It could also be a perfect way to finish off a ponytail combined with other types of braids such as the 2-Strand Twist.

Jamie's Law: When doing steps 2 and 4, make sure you reach *behind* the free hanging section. If you take the sections from the top, it will not wrap around the sides and the finished look will be affected.

1. Divide ponytail into two sections.

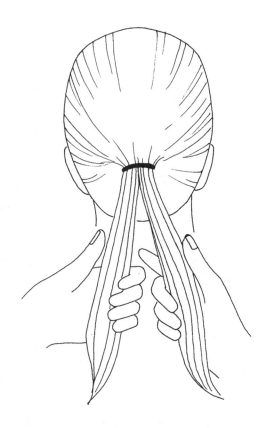

2. Take a small section from behind the left side section.

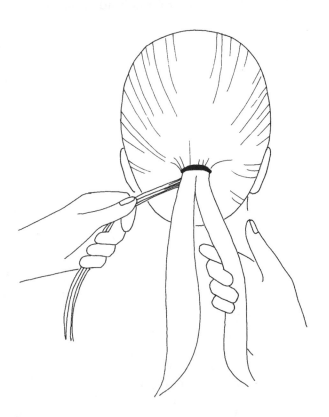

3. Give it to the right side.

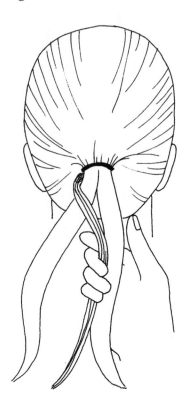

4. While holding ponytail securely with the left thumb, and allowing the right side to hang free, take a small section from behind the right side.

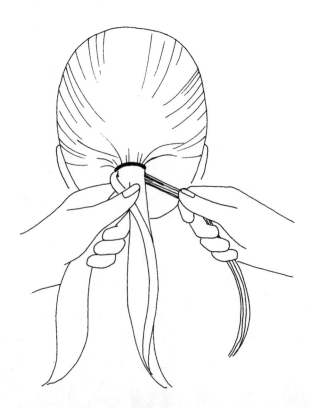

5. Give it to the left side.

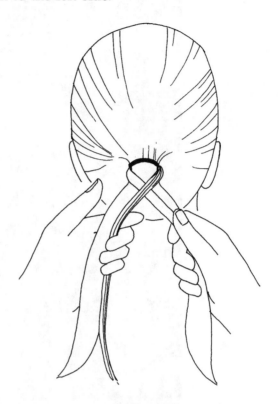

6. While holding the right side securely with your right thumb, continue steps 2 through 6 until you reach the end of the ponytail. Secure with a rubberband.

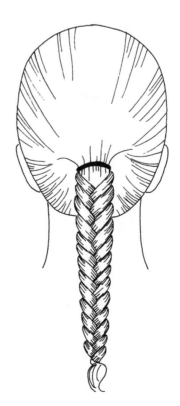

STYLE 7

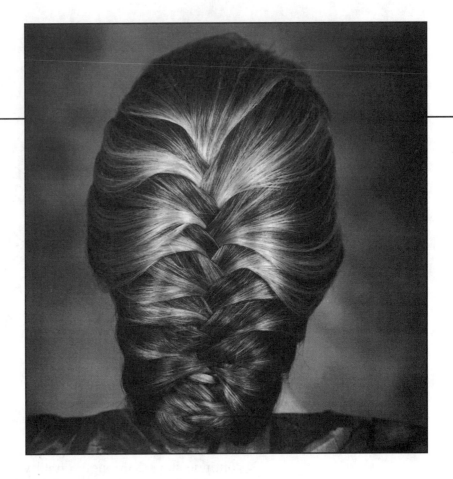

Fishtail

We are going to take the technique you learned in the Fishtail Ponytail and add to it to create the Fishtail Braid that starts in the bang area. If you have perfected the ponytail technique, you will be doing this one in no time at all. The fishtail is best done on dry, non-layered hair, shoulder length or longer. It is guaranteed to be one of your favorites.

Jamie's Law: Make an X. When you pick up one side, make sure you give it to the side opposite from the one you picked up on.

1. Take a triangle section of hair from the front. If there are bangs, begin behind them.

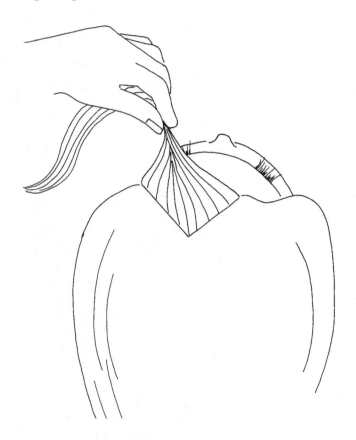

2. Divide this section into two strands.

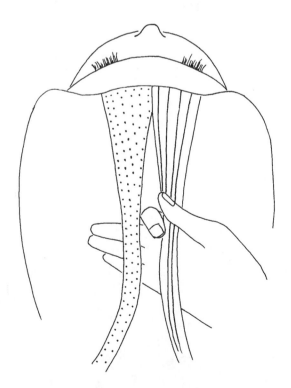

3. Cross the right strand over the left strand.

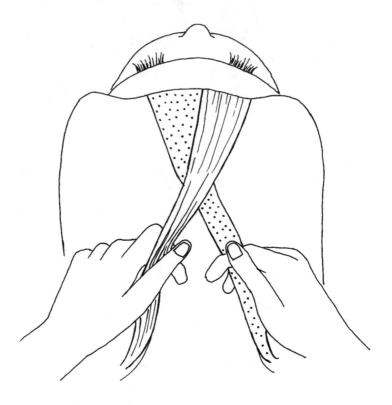

4. Place both strands in the right hand with the index finger inbetween, palm up, as shown.

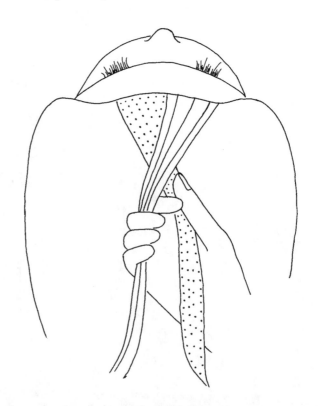

5. Pick up a 1" section on the left side. Starting at the hairline, continue across the head and end in the middle by your right hand.

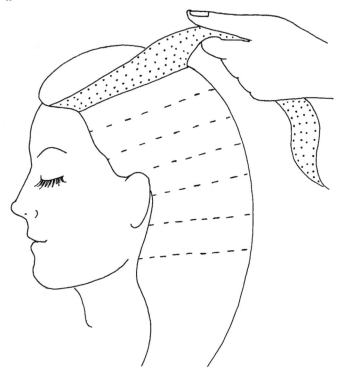

6. Cross this section over the left strand and add to the right strand. (Makes one side of an X.)

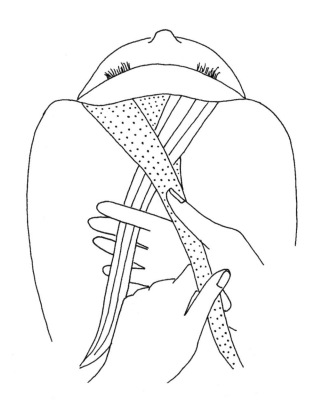

7. Put both strands in the left hand with the index finger inbetween, palm up, as shown.

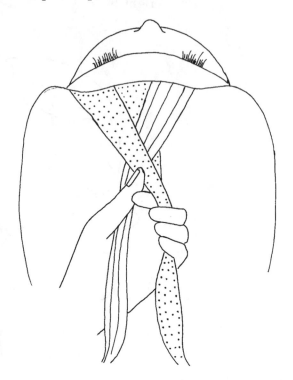

8. Pick up a 1" section on the right side. Starting at the hairline, continue across the head and end in the middle by your left hand.

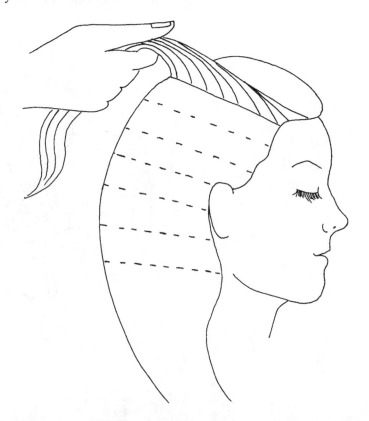

9. Cross the section over the right strand and add it to the left strand. (Makes the other side of an X.)

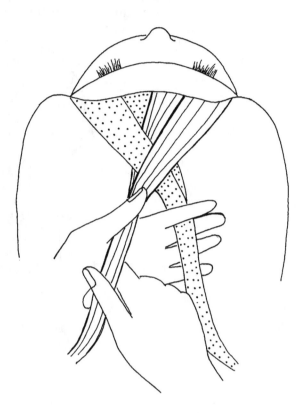

10. Put both strands in the right hand with index finger in-between, palm up, as shown.

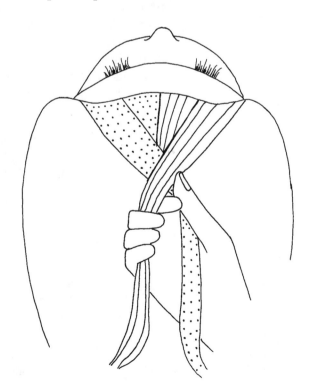

11. Repeat steps 5 through 10, allowing your hand to move down to the nape with each 1" section picked up. When you run out of sections, secure with a rubberband.

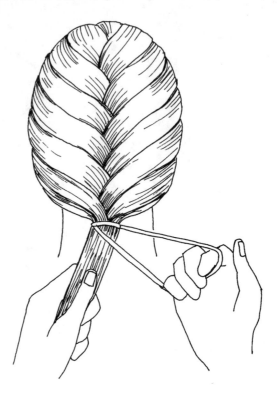

12. Another option would be to keep your hands elevated at crown level while you are doing this braid. Once finished, but before you put the rubberband in the hair, let your hands relax to the nape area and allow the braid to slide down. This technique creates fullness behind the ears. Finish off the ponytail with the fishtail ponytail technique, then tuck under and secure with bobbypins. The finished style will look like this.

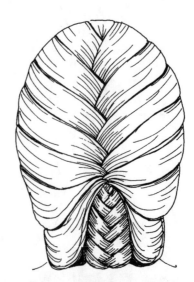

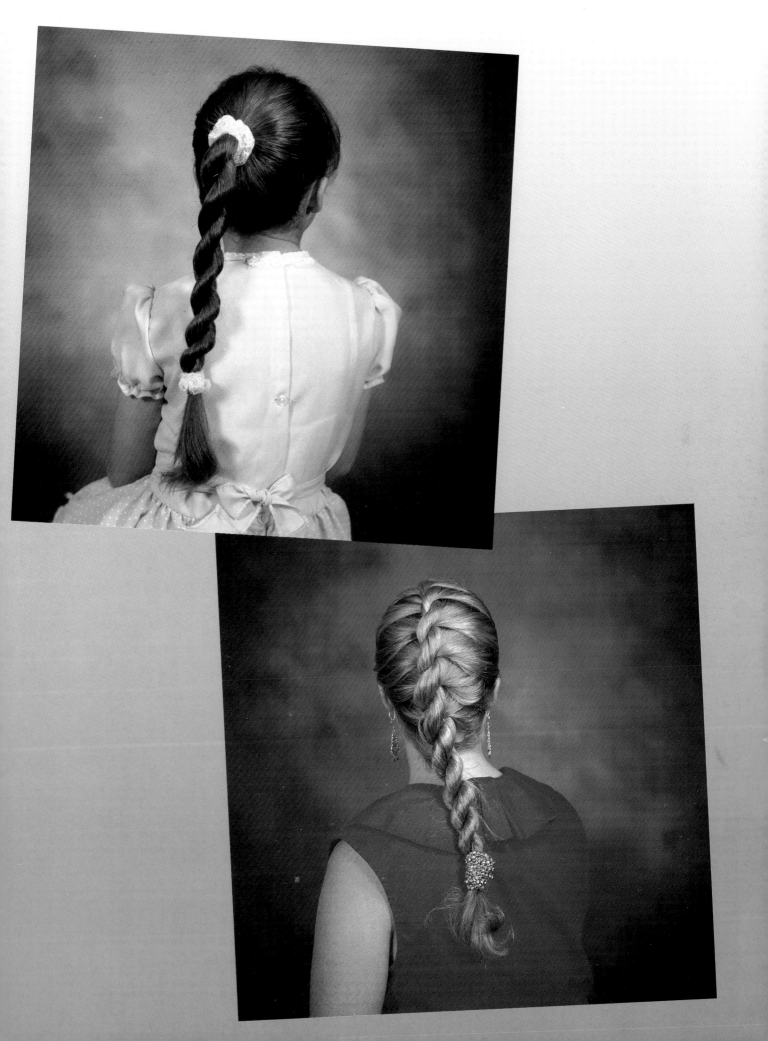

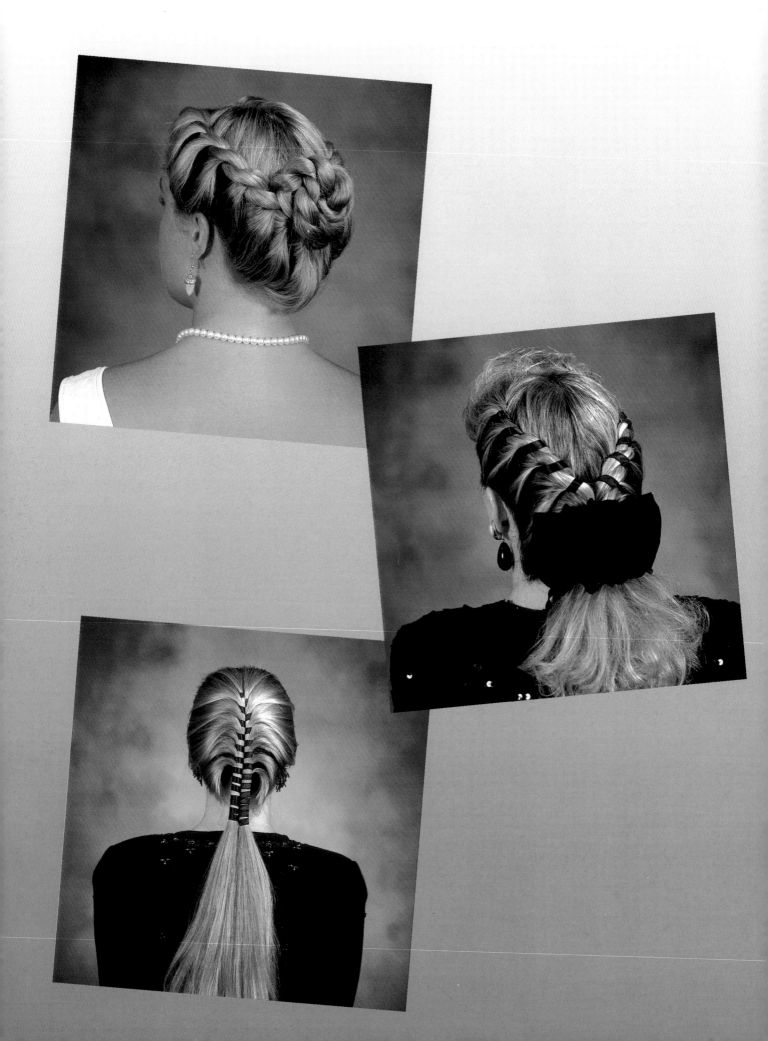

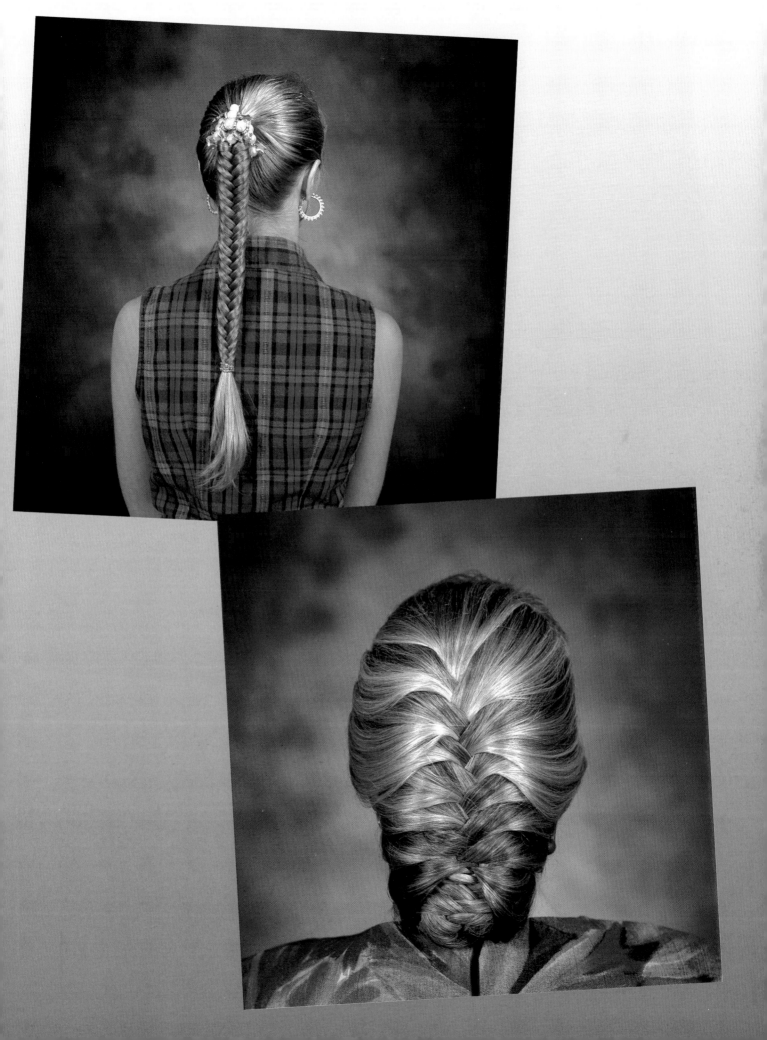

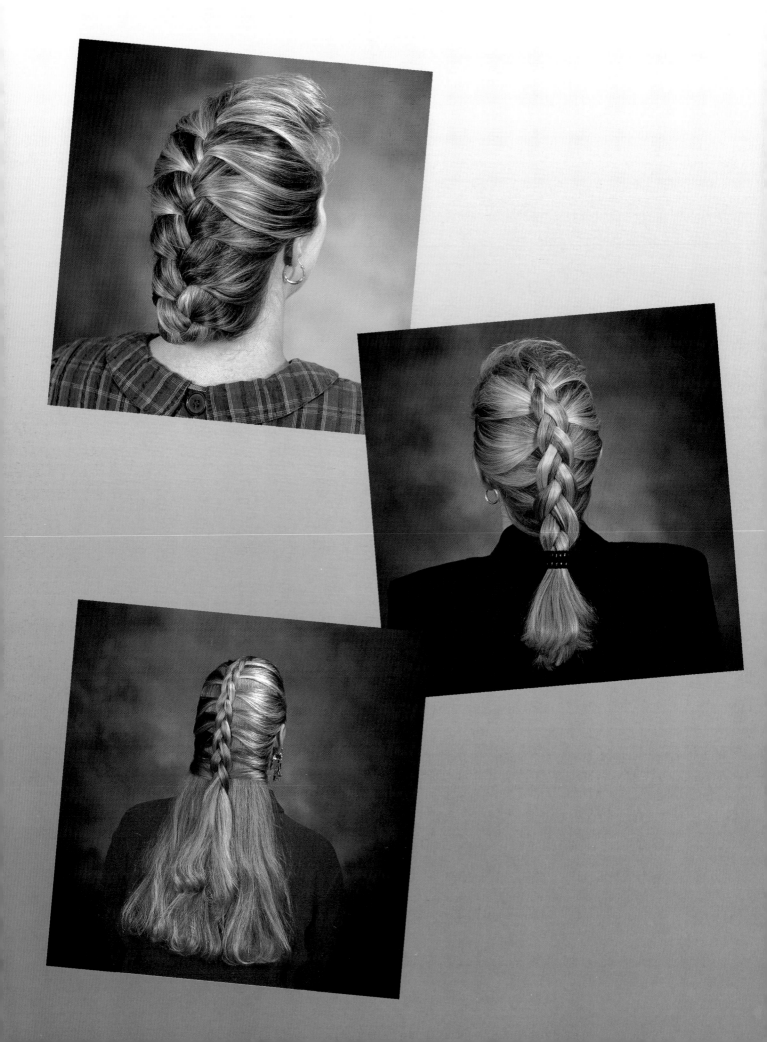

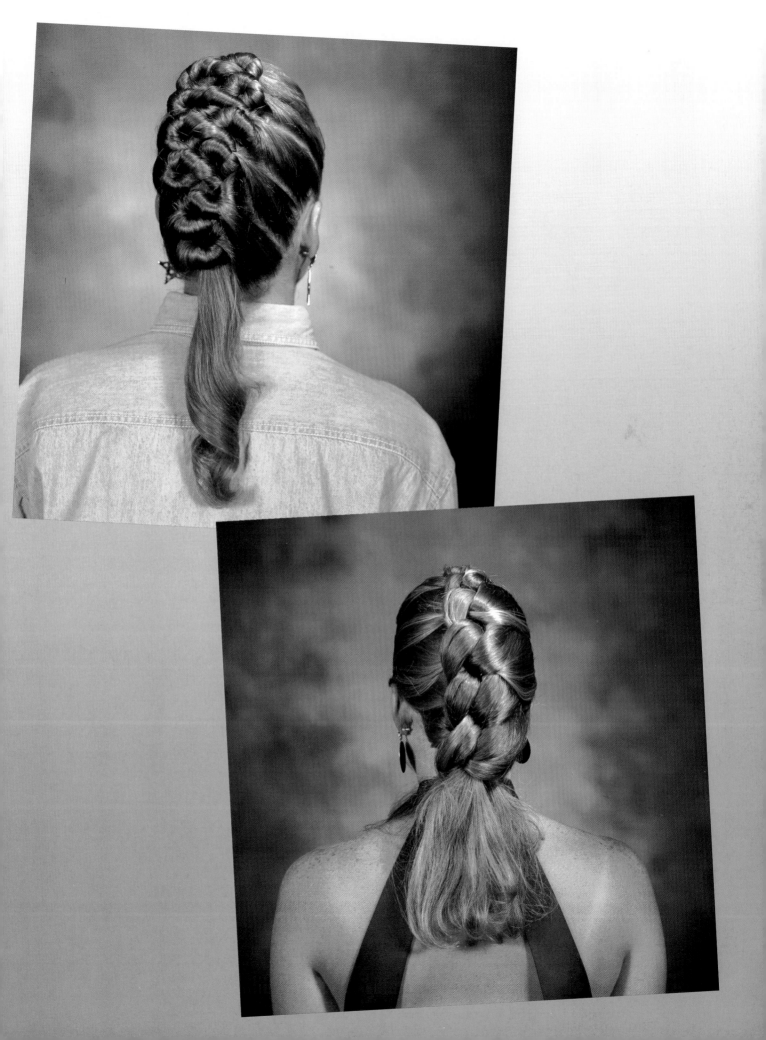

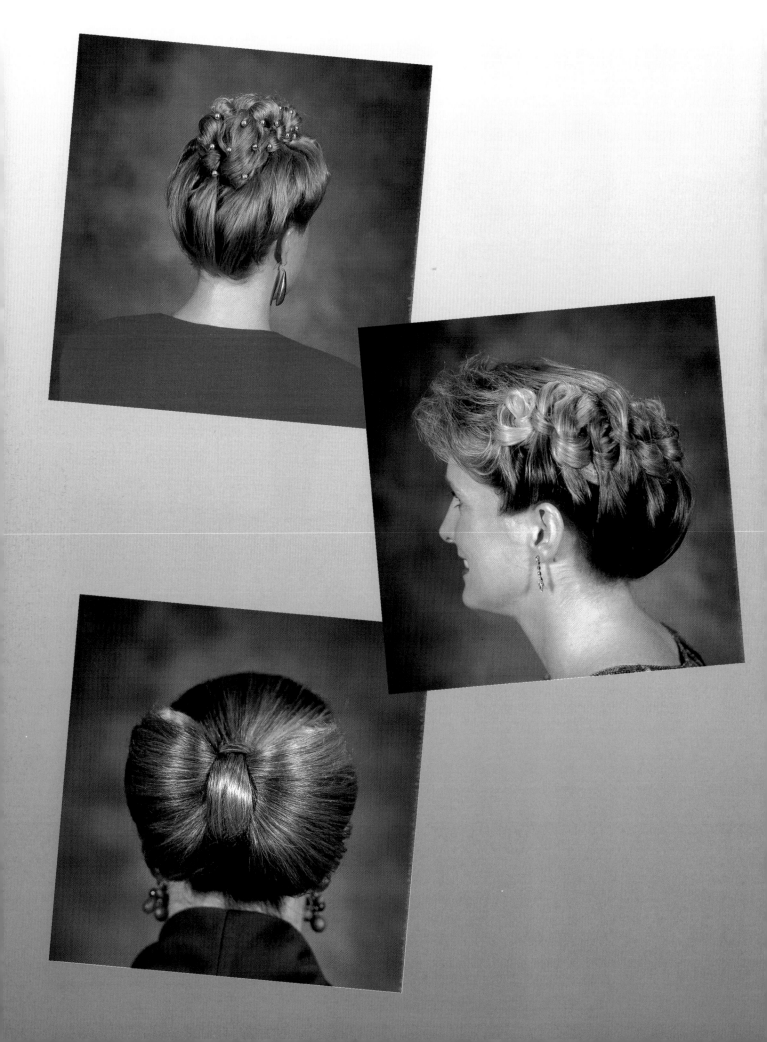

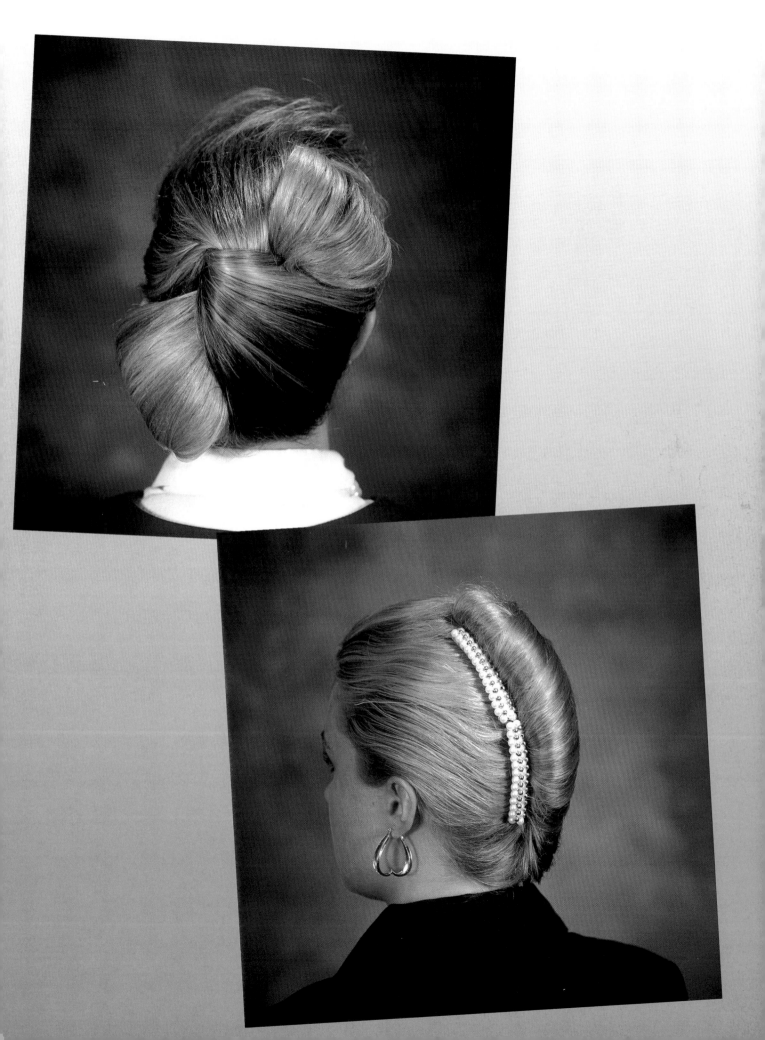

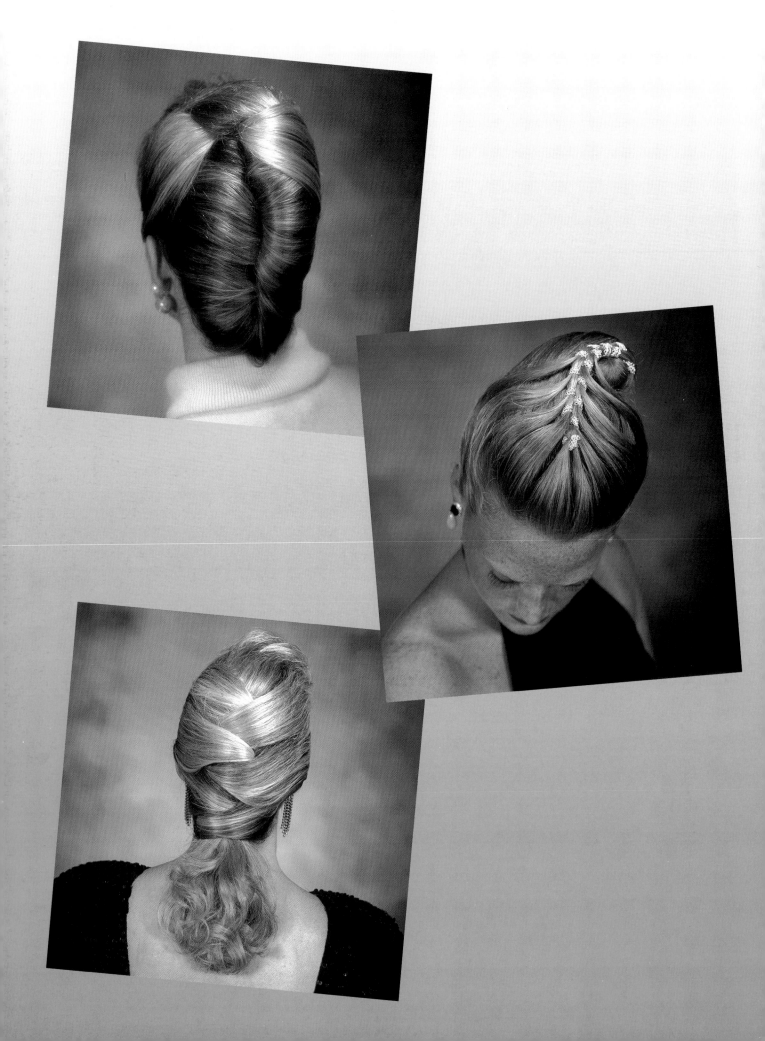

STYLE 8

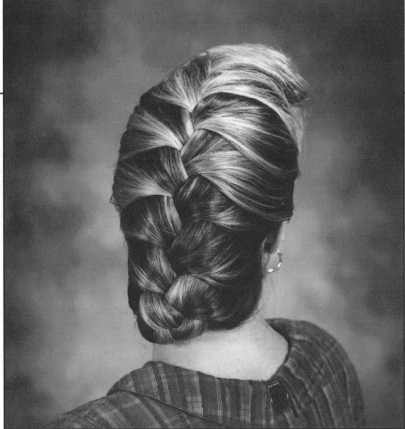

French Braid

We are now beginning the 3-strand braids. To make them easier to learn, pay special attention to the hand positions, and copy them exactly. This will take the confusion out of working with three strands of hair at one time.

Once you have perfected the 3-strand techniques, you are unlimited by the amount of different styles you can create. By varying the direction or the amount of braids, you can create completely different looks. For example, put a French Braid on the left side and then one on the right side. Rubberband together with a ponytail hanging in the back. Or try doing a Dutch Braid but start it in the nape area instead of the bang area. You are truly unlimited in the different styles you can create once you know these braids.

The French Braid is the most requested braid in the salon and is always in style. It can be done on layered or all one-length hair. If done on layered hair, it is best to dampen and gel hair before braiding. If done on all one-length hair it is best done dry.

Jamie's Law: The French Braid is done by passing the outside strands *over* the center strands.

1. Take a triangle section of hair from the front. If there are bangs, begin behind them.

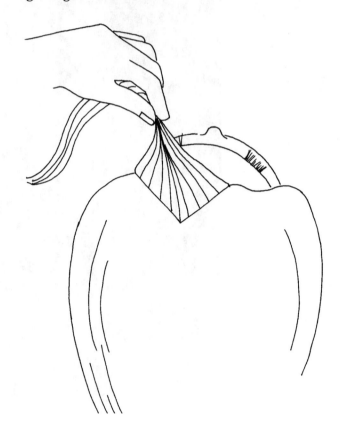

2. Divide this section into three strands.

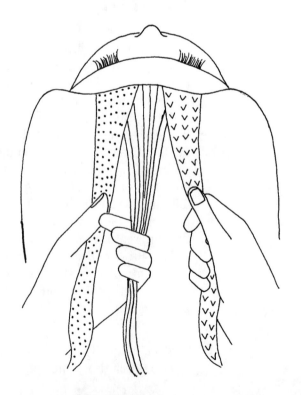

3. Cross the right strand over the center strand.

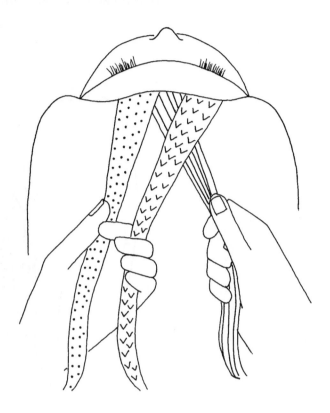

4. Cross the left strand over the center strand.

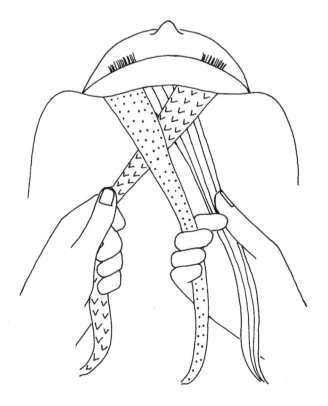

5. Place all three strands into left hand, with a finger in-between each section, palm up, as shown.

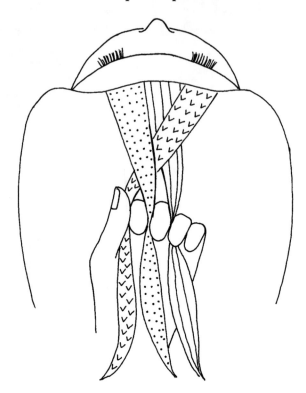

6. Pick up a 1" section on the right side.

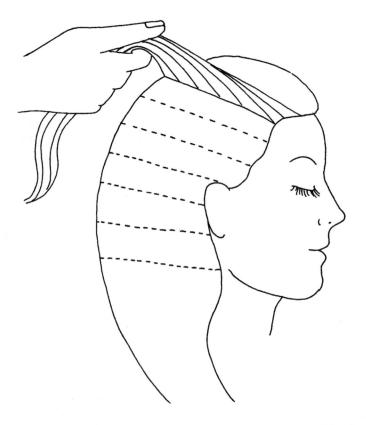

7. Add this section to the right strand already in your hand.

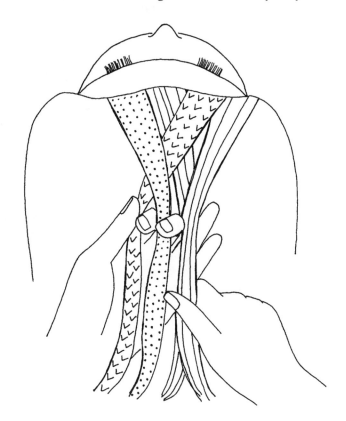

8. Cross right strand over center.

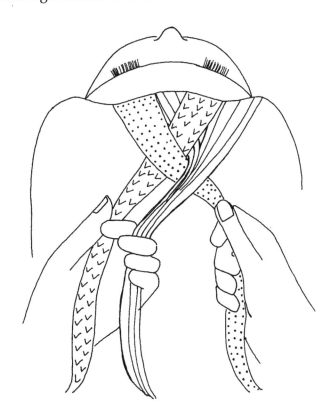

9. Place strands in right hand, fingers inbetween, palm up, as shown.

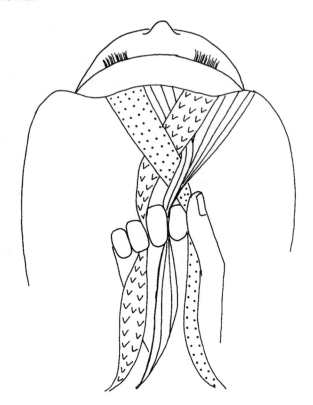

10. Pick up a 1" section on the left side.

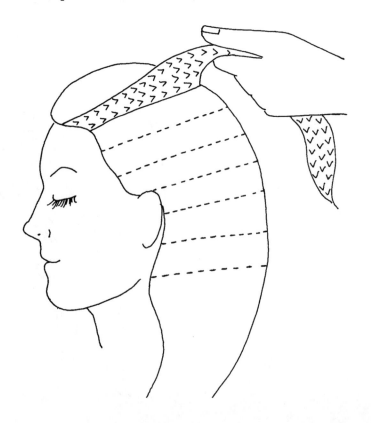

11. Add this section to the left strand already in your hand.

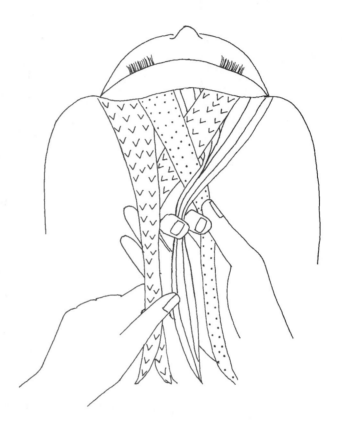

12. Cross the left strand over center strand.

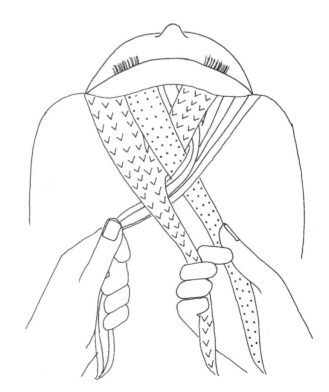

13. Place strands in left hand, fingers inbetween, palm up, as shown.

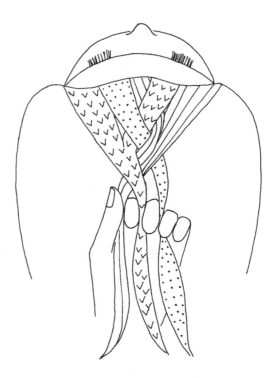

14. Repeat steps 6 through 13 moving down the nape with each 1" section picked up. When you run out of section, secure with rubberband. Remainder of hair forms ponytail.

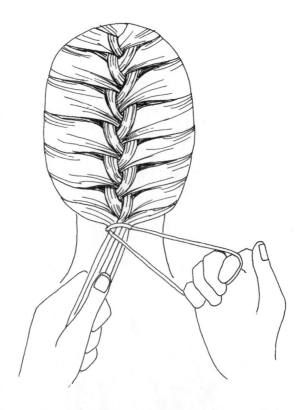

15. Or finish the ponytail by braiding to the ends, as shown.

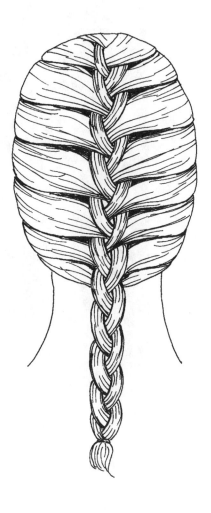

STYLE 9

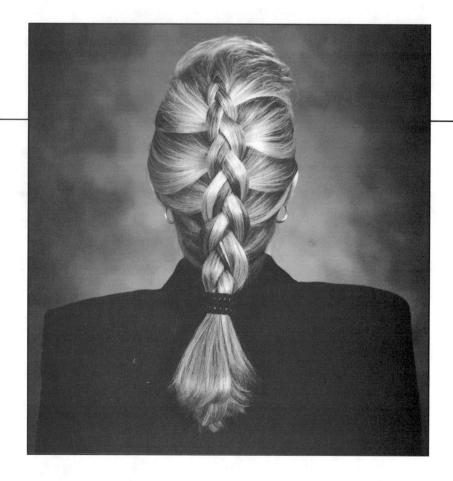

Dutch Braid

The Dutch Braid is very similar to the French Braid. The major difference is that the Dutch Braid sits on top and the French Braid is hidden underneath. The technique is similar too. It differs only in that you pass the strands under the center sections instead of over. It can be done on layered or all one-length hair. If done on layered hair, it is best to dampen and gel hair before braiding. If done on all one-length hair, it is best done dry.

Jamie's Law: The Dutch Braid is done by crossing the outside strands *under* the center strands.

1. Take a triangle section of hair from the front. If there are bangs, begin behind them.

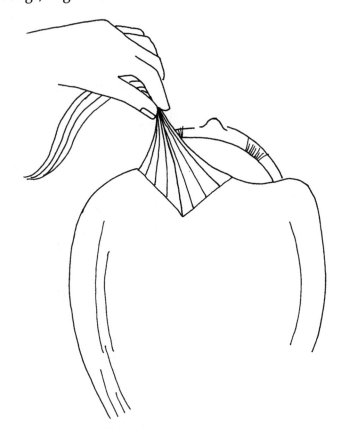

2. Divide this section into three strands.

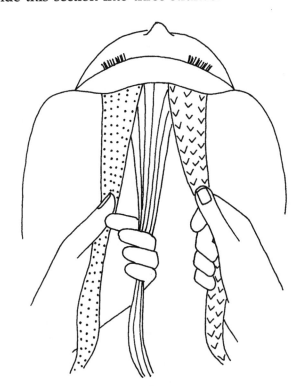

3. Cross the right strand under the center strand.

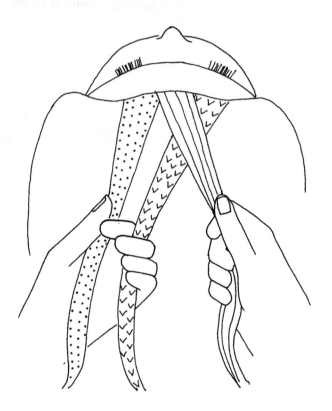

4. Cross the left strand under the center strand.

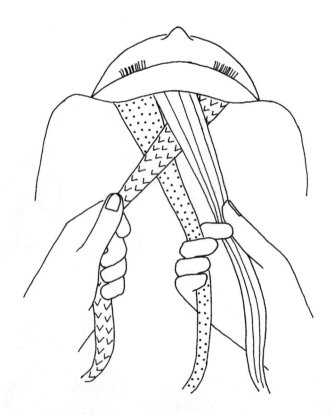

5. Place all three strands into left hand, with a finger between each section, palm up, as shown.

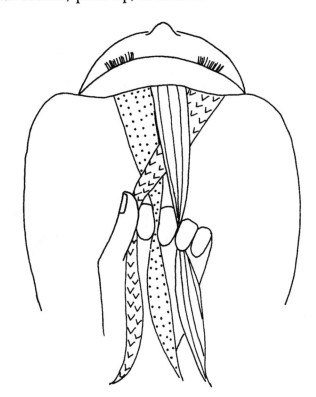

6. Pick up a 1" section on the right side.

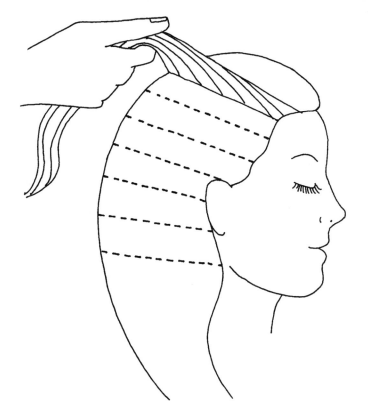

7. Add this section to the right strand already in your hand.

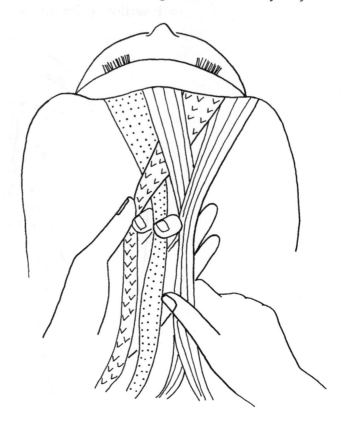

8. Cross right strand under center.

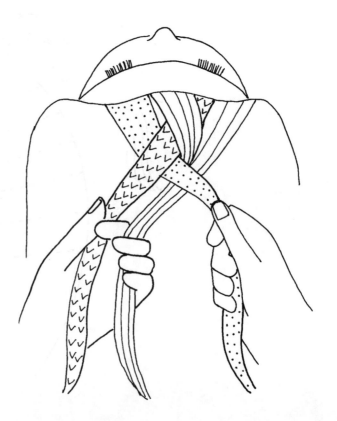

9. Place strands in right hand, fingers inbetween, palm up, as shown.

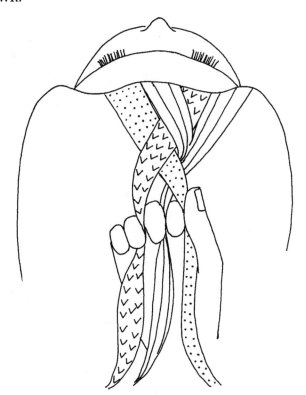

10. Pick up a 1" section on the left side.

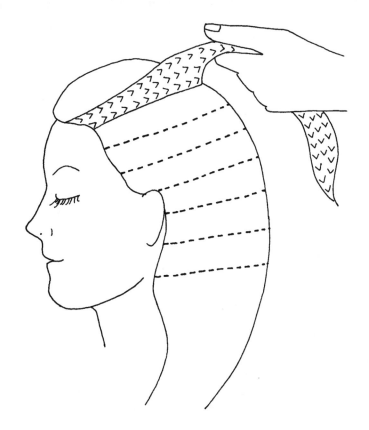

11. Add this section to the left strand already in your hand.

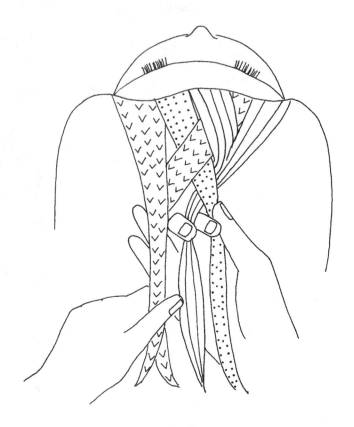

12. Cross the left strand under center strand.

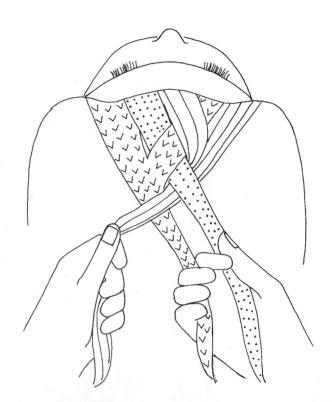

13. Place strands in left hand, fingers inbetween, palm up, as shown.

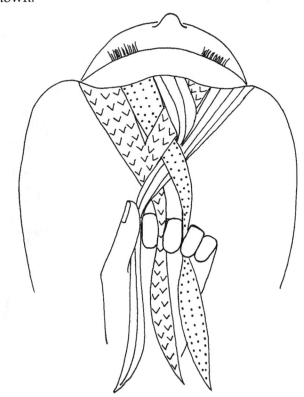

14. Repeat steps 6 through 13, moving down the nape with each 1" section picked up. When you run out of section, secure with rubberband. Remainder of hair forms ponytail.

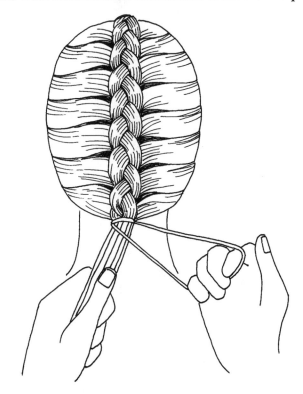

15. Or finish the ponytail by braiding to the ends, as shown.

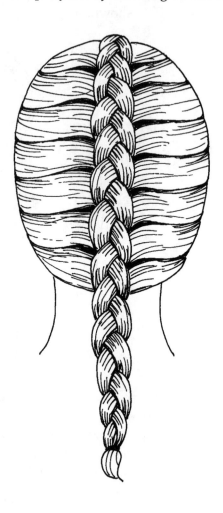

STYLE 10

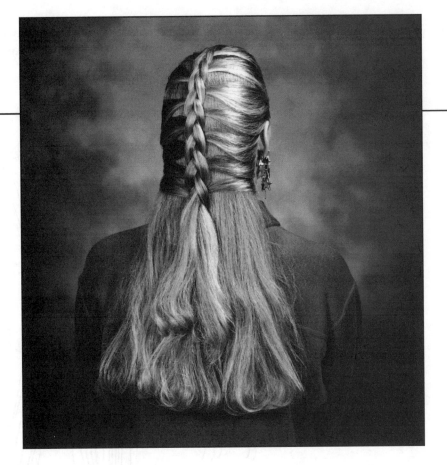

Hairline Dutch Braid

Now that you have perfected the Dutch Braid, try this version. You will find this style used quite often in the salon. Once you learn this hairline technique, feel free to use different braids such as the Ribbon Braid instead of always using the Dutch Braid. This style is best done on dry, all one-length hair.

Jamie's Law: You will braid only the hairline hair.

1. Make a 2" section of hair all the way around the hairline on both sides. Comb all other hair back into a ponytail and secure with a rubberband.

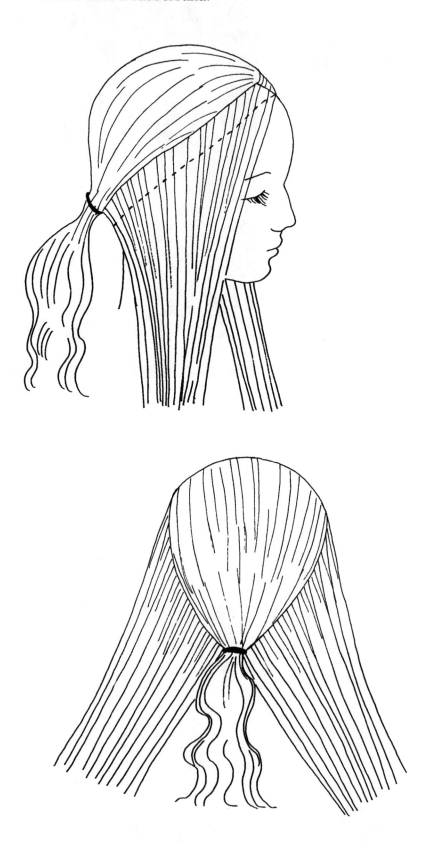

2. Take a 3" section of hairline hair in the bang area as shown. Divide this section into three strands.

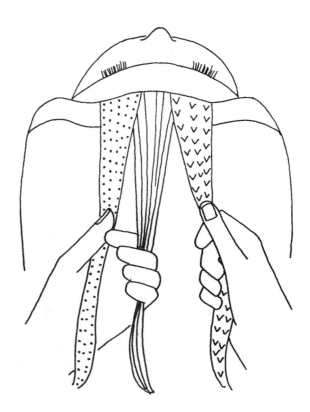

3. Cross the right strand under the center strand.

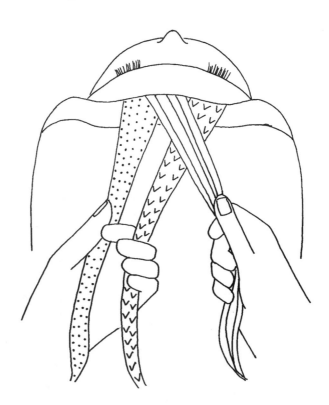

4. Cross the left strand under the center strand.

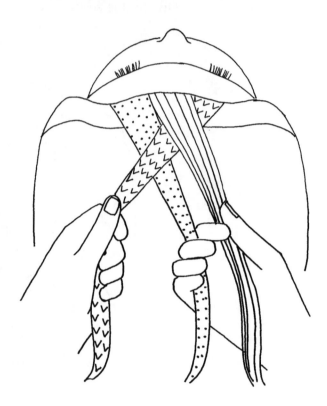

5. Place all three strands into the left hand, with a finger between each section, palm up, as shown.

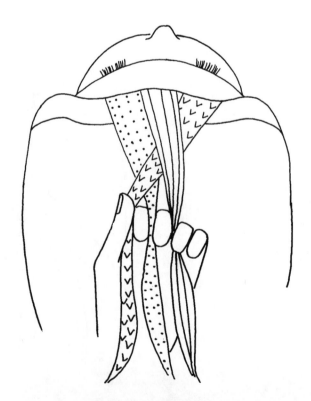

6. Pick up a 1" section on the right side.

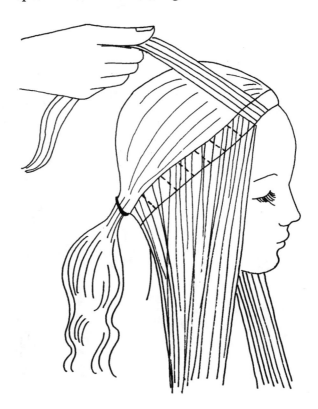

7. Add this section to the right side strand already in your hand.

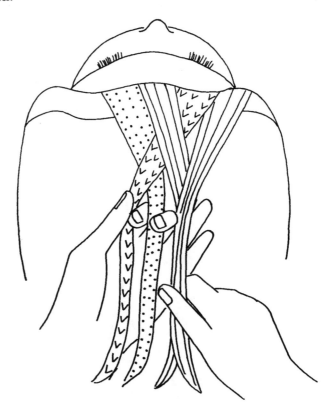

8. Cross right strand under center strand.

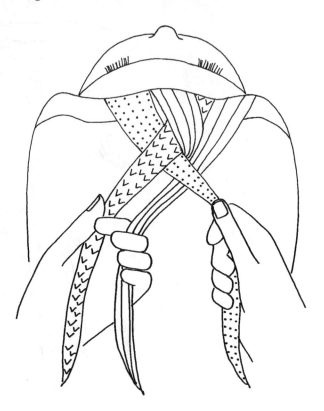

9. Place strands in right hand, fingers inbetween, palm up, as shown.

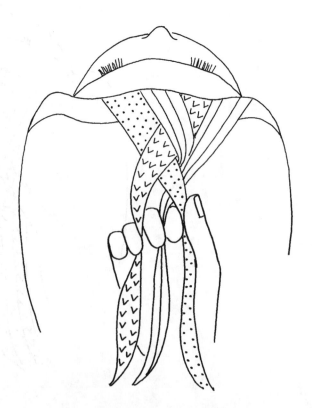

10. Pick up 1" section on the left side.

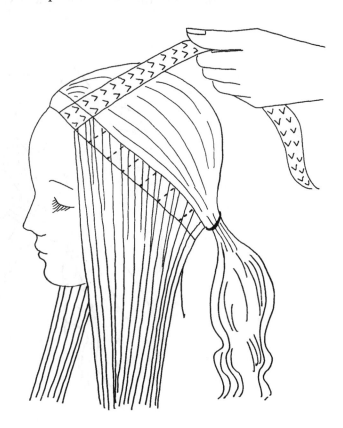

11. Add this section to the left strand already in your hand.

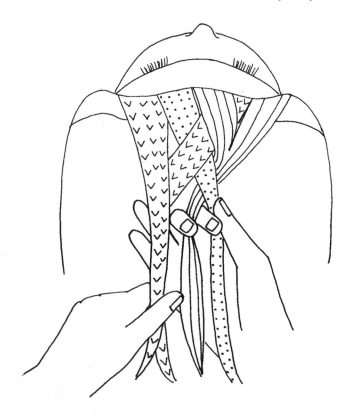

12. Cross the left strand under center strand.

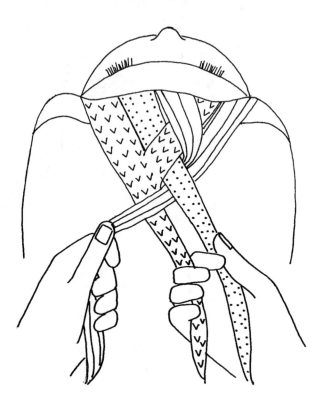

13. Place strand in left hand, fingers inbetween, palm up, as shown.

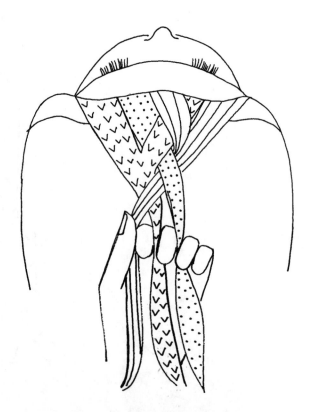

14. Repeat steps 6 through 13 moving down toward the nape with each section picked up. When you run out of section from the hairline, remove the rubberband and allow the other hair to fall free. Secure the braid with a bow. The braid acts like a net over the free hair underneath.

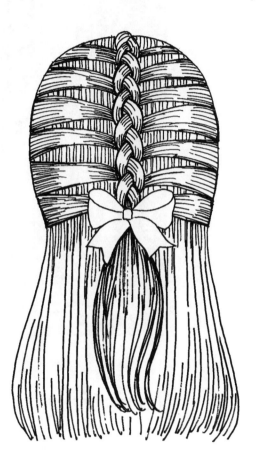

STYLE 11

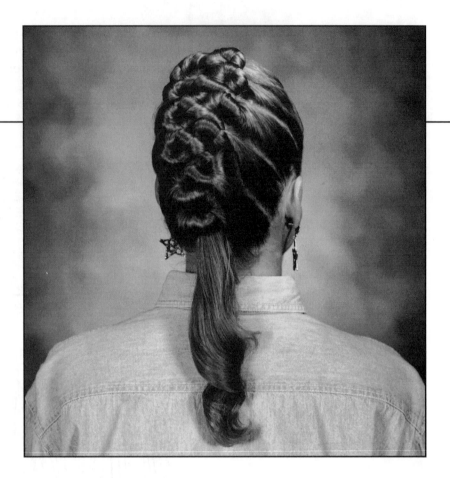

Twisting

The twisting techniques shown here can be as varied as the stylist doing them. Following are instructions for forming the twisted design into many figure-eights. But don't think this is the only way to do them. It is also very beautiful to allow the twist to be free form and lay where it may.

Jamies Law: Be certain the 1" section you are picking up passes over the existing strand, not under it.

1. Take a triangle section just to the left side of center. If there are bangs, begin behind them.

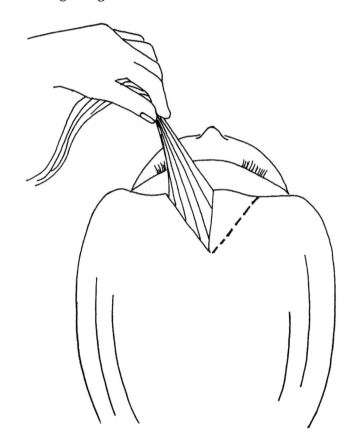

2. Begin twisting this section of hair toward the right, and move your body over by your client's right shoulder.

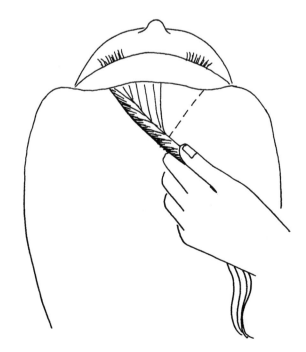

3. Pick up a 1" section on the right side.

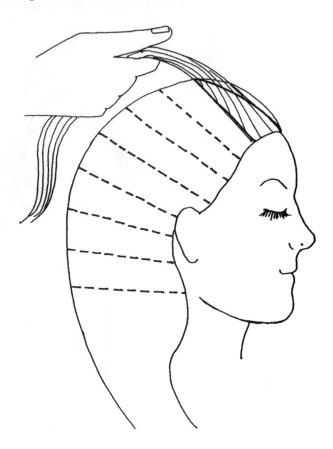

4. Take this new strand and pass it over the top of the twisted strand.

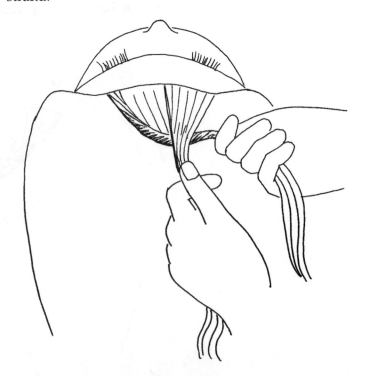

5. Continue wrapping this new strand in a counterclockwise direction around the twisted strand until they become one strand.

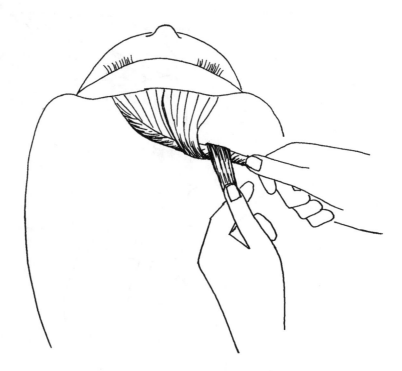

6. As you walk to your client's left shoulder, force the twisted strand up to form the top part of an eight.

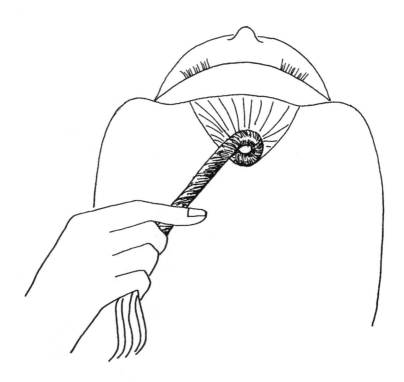

7. Pick up a 1" section on the left side.

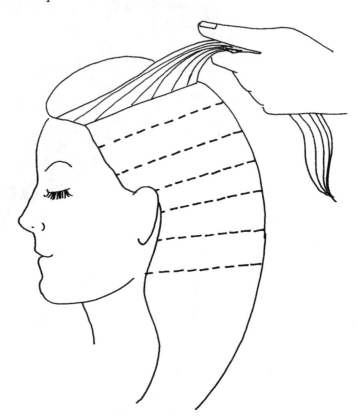

8. Take this new strand and pass it over the top of the twisted strand.

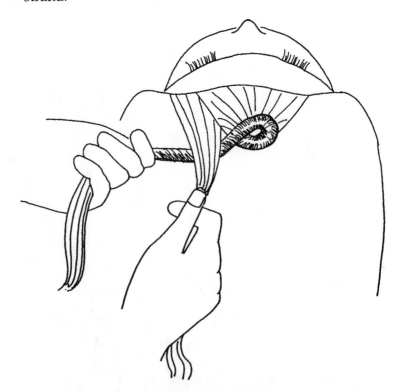

9. Continue wrapping this new strand in a clockwise direction around the twisted strand until they make one strand.

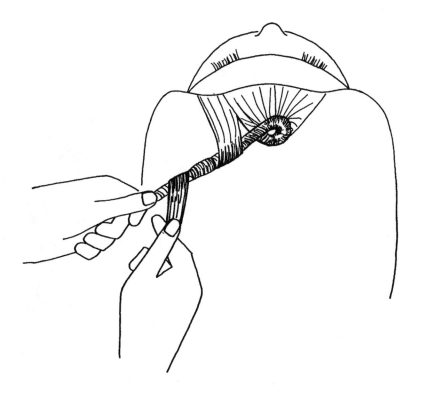

10. As you walk to your client's right shoulder, force the twisted strand up to form the bottom part of an eight.

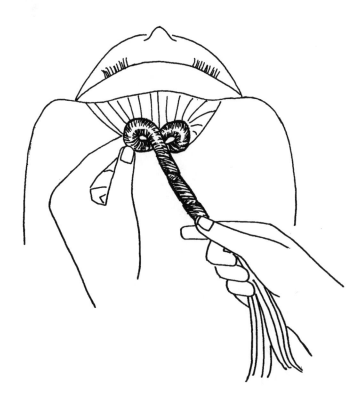

11. Repeat steps 3 through 10, moving down toward the nape with each 1" section picked up. When you run out of sections, secure with bobbypins. You might want to softly curl the piece of remaining hair and place it over the client's shoulder.

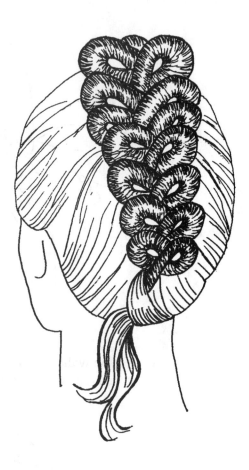

STYLE 12

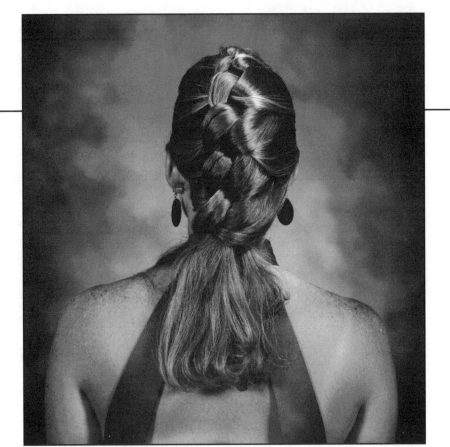

Knotting

This updo is easy and fun to do. People always ask how it's done because it looks so complicated. But, as you have already learned, just because you can't figure out how it's done by looking at it doesn't mean it is difficult to do. The key to knotting is that it's best done on dry, all one-length hair.

Jamie's Law: You must tie the knots exactly the same each time. If you tie right over left, as we have done here, you must follow through and tie it that way each time.

1. Make a triangle section at the top. If your client has bangs, begin behind them.

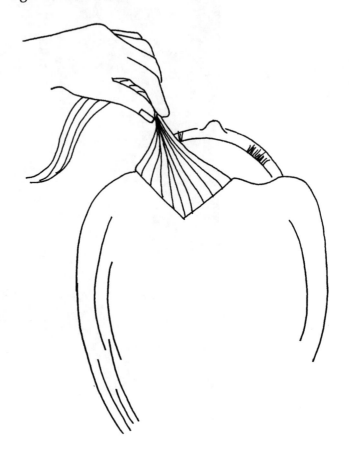

2. Divide this section into two strands.

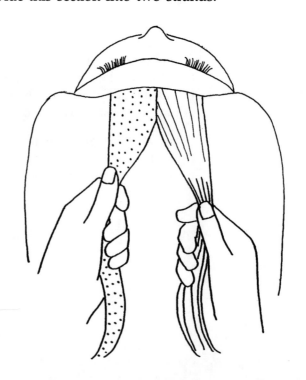

3. Place both sections in your left hand, matching the hand positions shown. Then, place the right strand over the left strand.

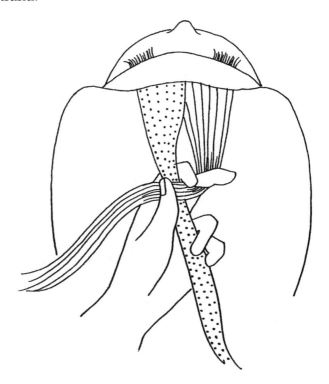

4. Using your right thumb and index fingers, reach between the strands and pull the right strand through the two strands.

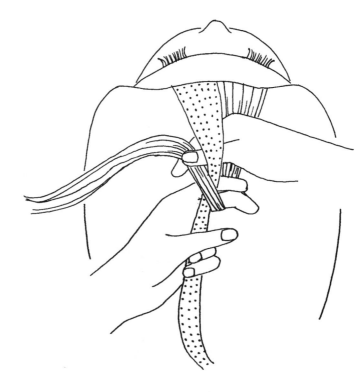

5. Make sure the strand you pulled between the two strands is kept to the left side.

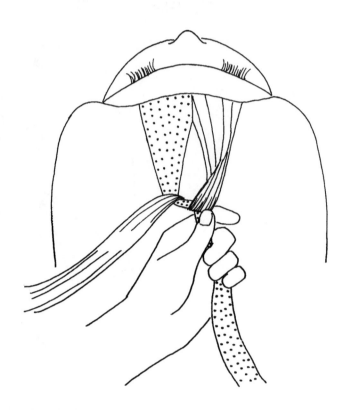

6. Pull both strands so the hair ties next to the scalp. You have just tied the first part of a knot.

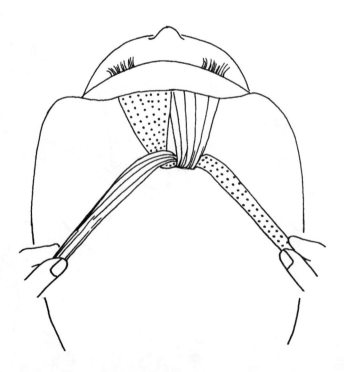

7. Place both strands in the left hand, fingers inbetween. Pick up a 1" section on the right side of the head.

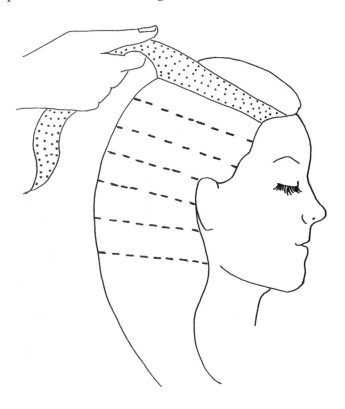

8. Add this section to the right side section already in your hand.

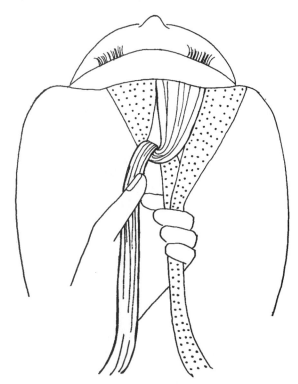

9. Place both sections in your right hand, finger inbetween as shown. (You have just changed hands).

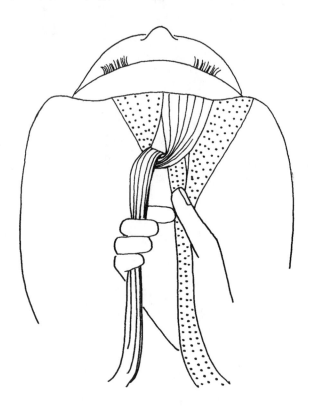

10. Pick up a 1" section on the left side of the head.

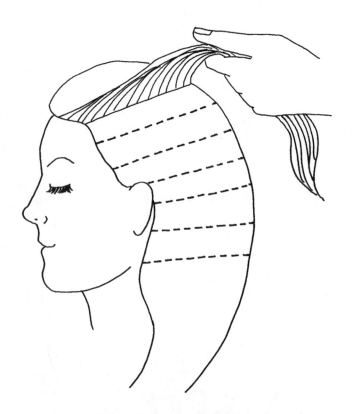

11. Add it to the left side section already in your hand.

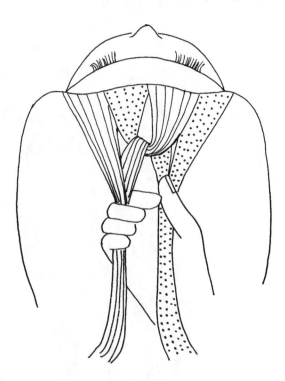

12. Repeat steps 3 through 11, picking up 1" sections as you move down the head. Continue until you reach the nape and run out of sections to pick up. Tie the two strands together a few more times, then roll under and pin. Curl remaining tendrals with a curling iron and rest over shoulder.

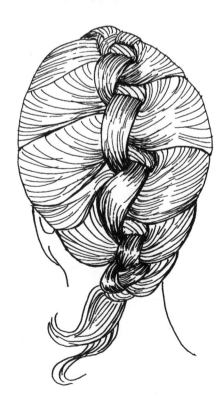

STYLE 13

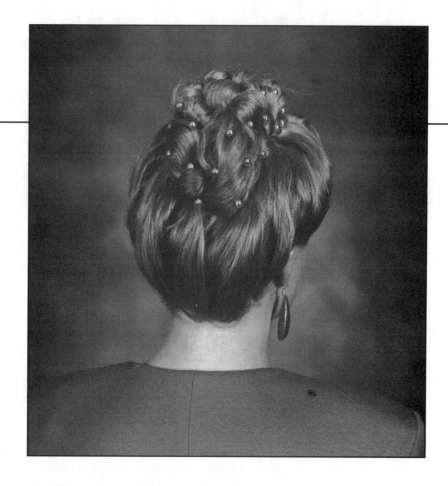

Looping on Top

Looping is a simple technique that creates fullness without backcombing or setting. It can be done on straight or curly hair as well as long, layered or all one-length hair. There is no need to prepare the hair with any gels. Just begin on clean dry hair and use hairspray when you're finished. This is a perfect updo to accessorize with gold beads on a hairpin. (see pages 19 through 20).

Jamie's Law: In order to create fullness, push the hair forward after you make the loop and before you secure with a bobby pin.

1. Pick up a triangle section in the bang area.

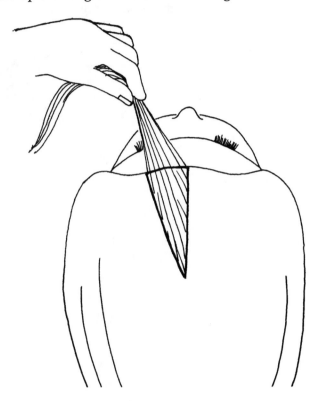

2. Wrap this section around your index and middle fingers on your left hand.

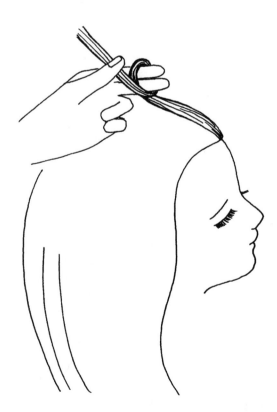

3. Using your right thumb and index fingers, reach through the loop and get the hair strand.

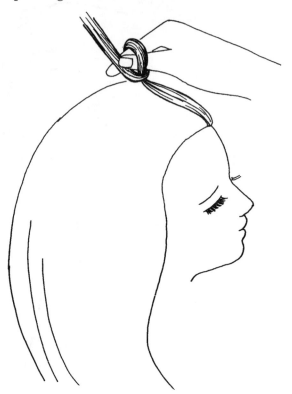

4. Pull it partly through as shown.

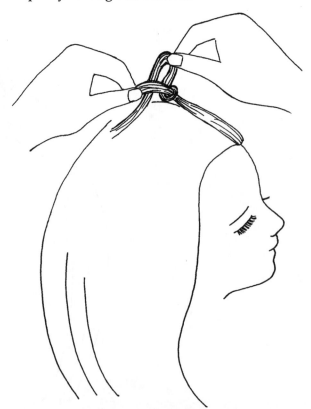

5. Holding the base of the loop, push this section forward to create fullness, then pin securely with a bobby pin. If the hair is very long, you can make another loop with the remainder of the hair strand, or you may leave the end of the strand against the head and place other loops on top of it to hide the ends.

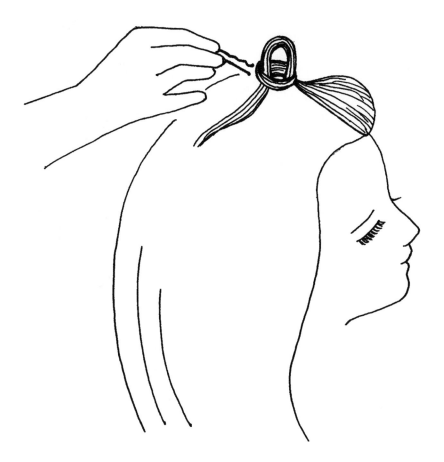

6. Make 1"-2" pivotal parting while working your way around the head. After completing the loop on each section, make sure you push each section forward to create fullness before you bobby pin.

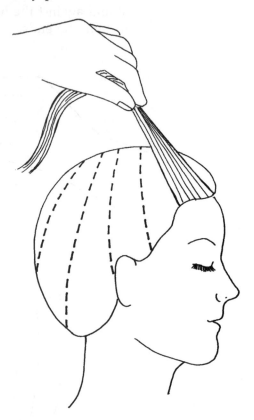

7. Be creative when it comes to placing the loops. You can put them all on top, or do something different by placing them to the side or even the back of the head.

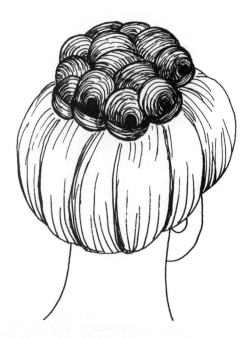

STYLE 14

Looping on Sides

This technique is done the same way as Looping on the Top (Chapter 23) except we are creating fullness on the sides instead of the top. There is no setting or back combing. Just section the hair, pin, and begin. Looping can be done on all one-length as well as long layered hair. It is just as beautiful on straight hair as it is on wavy hair.

Jamie's Law: Make sure bobby pins overlap each other as shown in step 1. Pay particular attention to doing this step securely since the entire style is attached to this bobby pin base.

1. Section the hair as shown. Leave out a triangle section in the bang area. Comb the remaining hair straight down. Leaving out a 1" section in front of both ears, begin by placing overlapping bobby pins around the head. Make sure you leave out a 1" section in front of both ears.

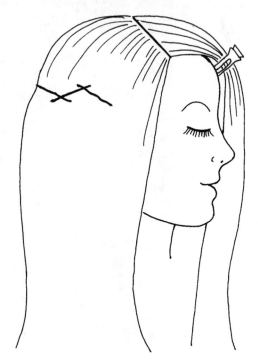

2. Take the front triangle section and comb back toward the crown.

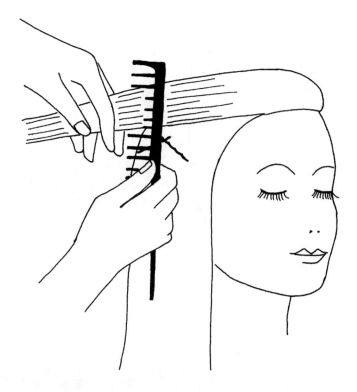

3. Holding the strand between your fingers, push forward toward the forehead until the hair falls into a wave.

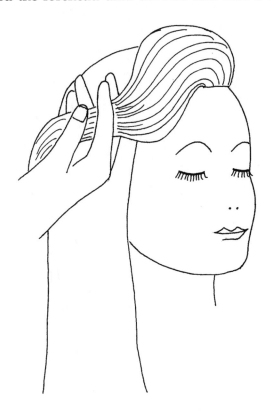

4. Bobby pin this section to the line of bobby pins previously placed.

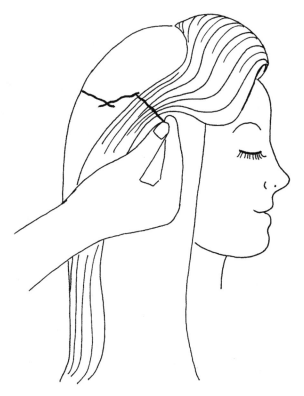

5. Clip this wave into place with a large clip until you have completed the looping.

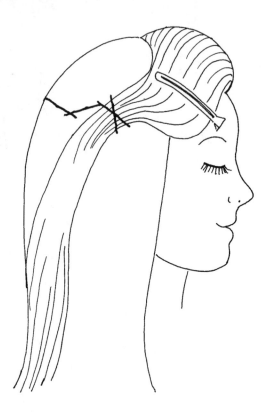

6. Pick up the 1" section that was not secured by bobby pins.

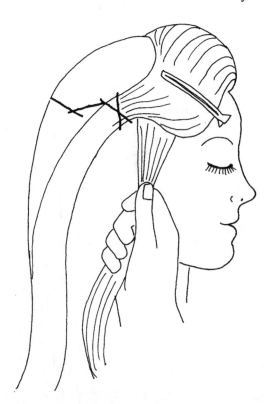

7. Wrap this section around the index and third fingers of your left hand and hold in place with your thumb as shown.

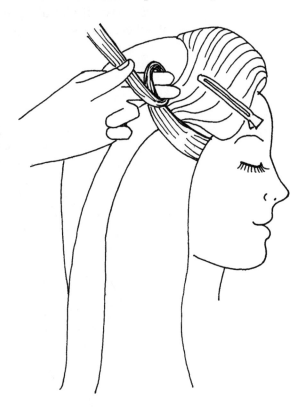

8. Reach through the loop with your thumb and index fingers.

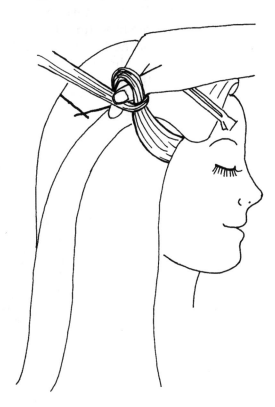

9. Pull the strand partially through the loop to form a curl. Secure the base with a bobby pin. Do not pin the loop or curl. Leave it standing upright and free, so you can place it where you want it to create curl or fullness.

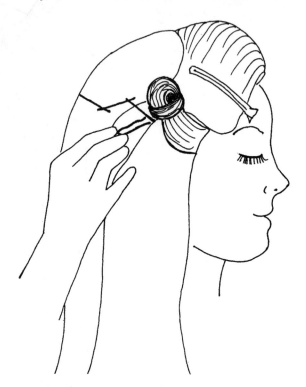

10. Continue forming curls while moving in 1" sections around the head until they are all completed. You can use the ends of the hair left over from the loops on long hair to create another loop or just pin the other loops on top to hide them.

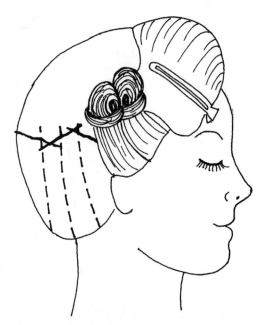

11. Finish with hairspray and remove large clip.

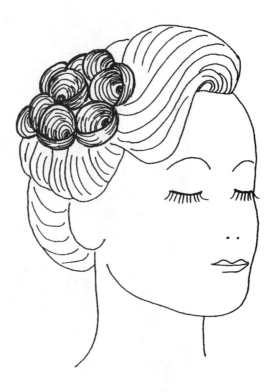

STYLE 15

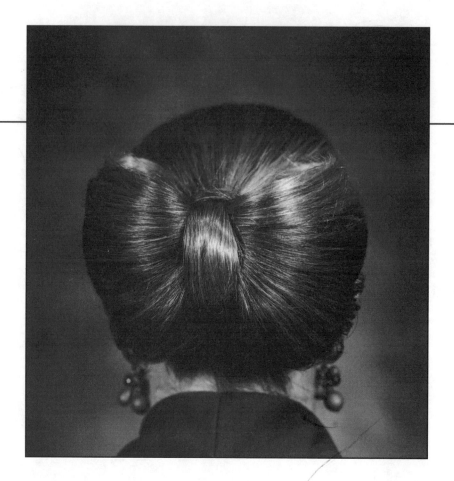

The Bow

Every stylist should know how to make a bow. It is such an elegant evening look. Following are instructions for making a bow very easily. See if you don't agree.

Jamie's Law: Be sure to cover the rubber band with hair or a hair accessory before you make the bow. It is too difficult to cover later.

1. Make a ponytail where you want the center of the bow to be positioned. Take a small section from underneath the ponytail and backcomb.

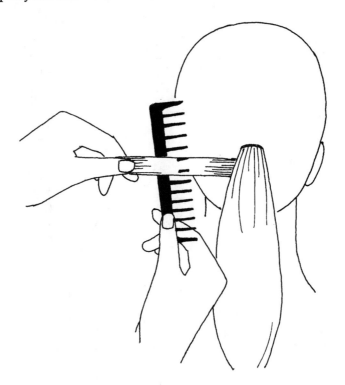

2. Wrap this backcombed section around rubber band and secure with hair pins.

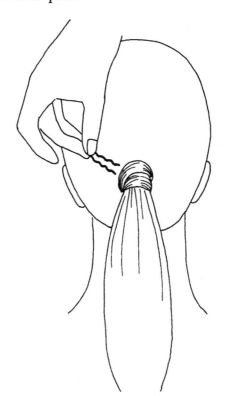

3. Remove a small section from the top of ponytail and clip up out of your way.

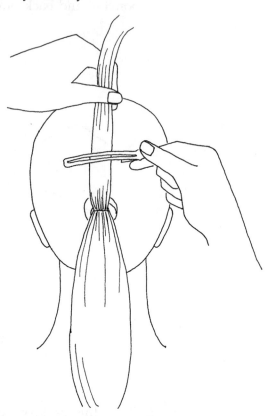

4. Divide remaining ponytail into two sections.

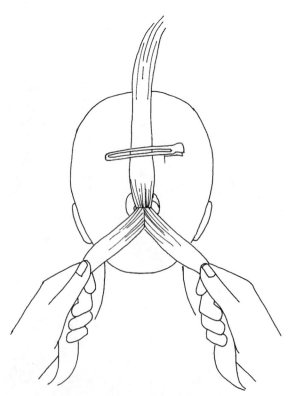

5. Clip left side out of your way. Backcomb the right side, making sure to hold hair straight out to the side as shown.

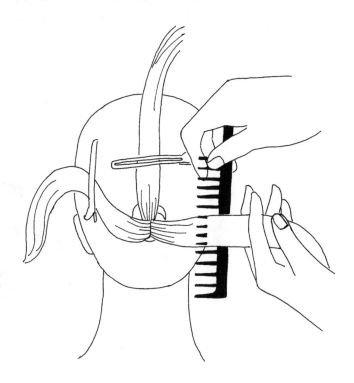

6. Roll backcombed section into a barrel curl placing it behind the right ear. Secure with bobby pins. Use your fingers to fan out barrel curl to make it as wide as possible without splitting. Use hairpins to tack in place. This is the finished right side of your bow.

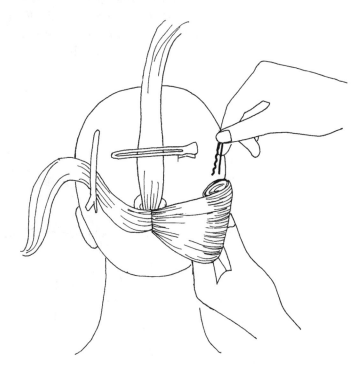

7. Next, backcomb left side and roll into a barrel curl placing it behind the left ear. Secure with bobby pins and fan out the barrel curl with your fingers making it as wide as possible.

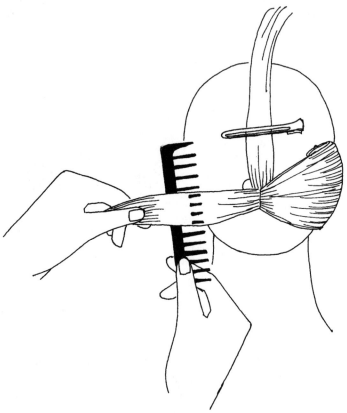

8. Take the small section you clipped out of your way in step 3 and gently back-comb. Roll this section into a pin curl. Lay this section over the split in the ponytail and bobby pin curl underneath.

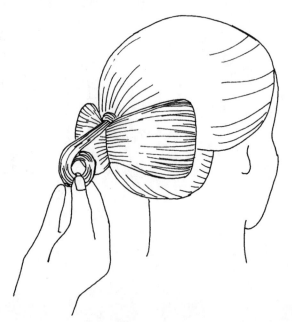

9. The finished bow will look like this. Make sure to use a finishing spray to keep smooth and fixed in place.

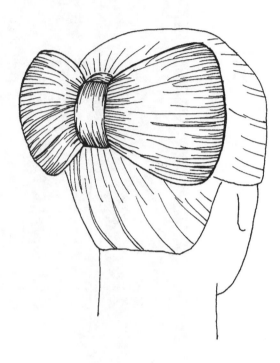

STYLE 16

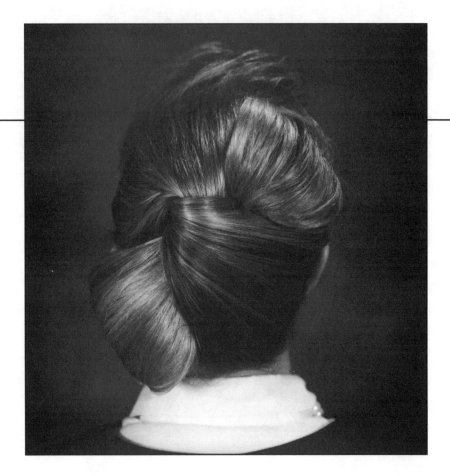

The Bowtie

The Bowtie is a beautiful finished style as well as a perfect base for many different long hair designs. It is recommended that you become comfortable tying this style, and then experiment with the ponytail pieces to create a completely different style. Have fun with the different options this style gives you.

The Bowtie is done best on dry, all one-length hair. When first learning how to tie this style you may find it easier to make it neat if you dampen and gel the hair first. This stops the strands from wrinkling when tied. If working with dampened hair backcombing is not recommended.

Jamie's Law: The right hand side must tie over, then under, the left side and end up at the crown.

1. Comb the hair back into a ponytail and hold it with your left hand. Using a tail comb, make a diagonal section along the scalp starting at the top of the right ear and ending behind the bottom of the left ear.

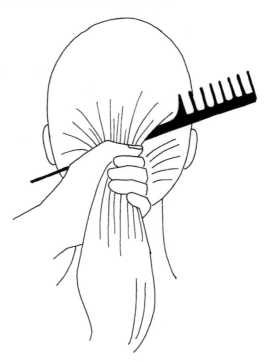

2. Put your comb down and place the right section in your right hand and the left section in your left hand.

   Hint: Try to copy the hand positions exactly on steps 3 and 4. This will take the confusion out of trying to manipulate these sections without the hair getting messy.

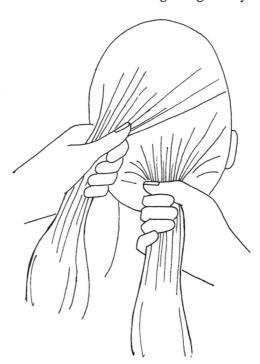

3. Using your thumb, index and third fingers to keep these sections separated, place the right section over the left section.

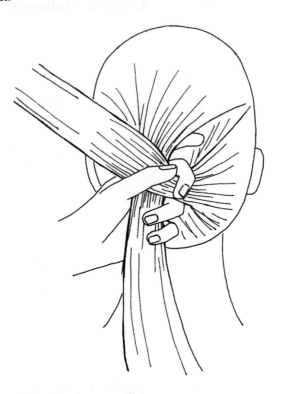

4. Reach through the strand separation and grab the strand on top. Pull it through and toward the crown.

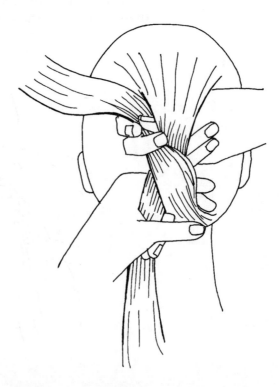

5. You have just tied the hair.

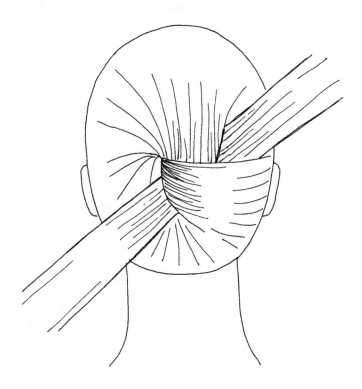

6. Using bobby pins make sure you securely fasten the tied section of the hair. This is very important. If not securely pinned the entire style can slide out.

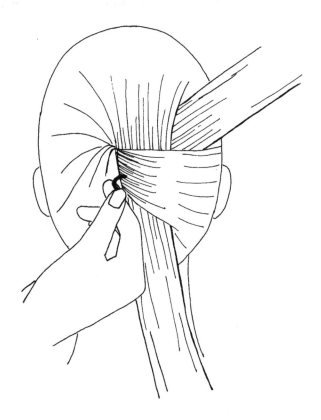

7. Using the section on the left, lightly backcomb it while directing the section behind the left ear.

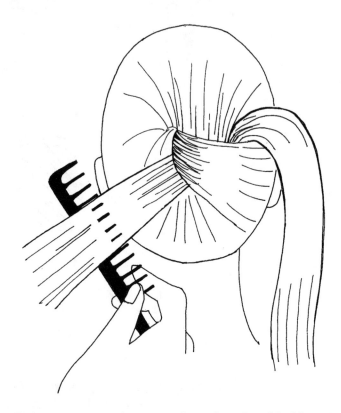

8. Roll this section under into a barrel curl and bobby pin into place. After pinning, spread this curl out as wide as you feel necessary.

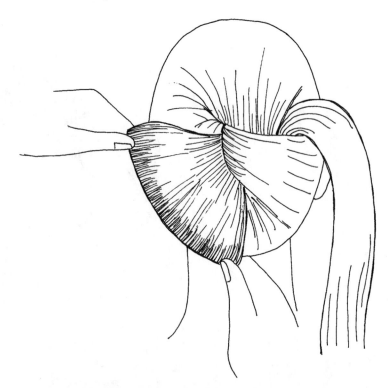

9. Lightly backcomb the top section, direct it forward toward the face and bobby pin as shown.

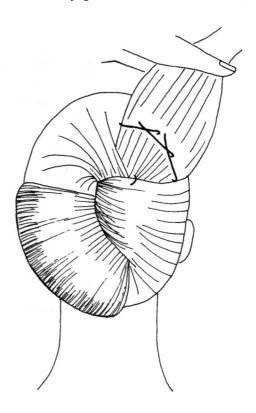

10. Make a barrel curl rolling back away from the face. Bobby pin this curl as close to the tied section as possible. Spread this curl as needed and use bobby pins to tack in place.

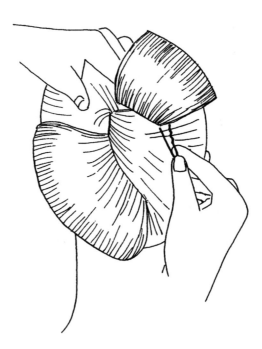

11. The finished style.

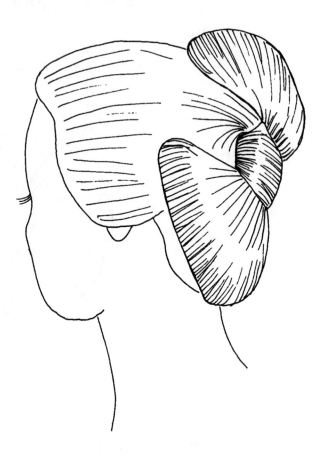

STYLE 17

French Twist

Following are instructions for the easiest way found to do the French Twist. There is no backcombing or any setting. It is a simple, smooth look with no fullness around the face. The technique will require practice, but once perfected you will use it often in the salon.

Jamie's Law: The hand positions are easily done when you stand in front of your client's right shoulder.

1. Comb the hair back into a ponytail and hold it with your left hand, palm facing toward nape with hand in a "V" position as shown.

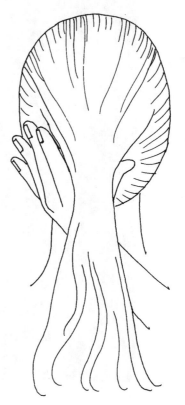

2. Close fingers together making sure to keep hand in the closed "V" position. Do not close hand into a circle as with a ponytail.

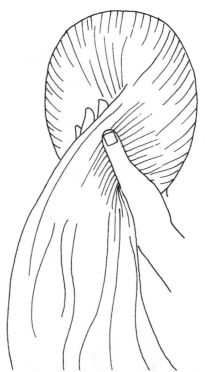

3. Reaching over your clients head with your right arm, grab the hair strand and begin twisting the entire strand to your right.

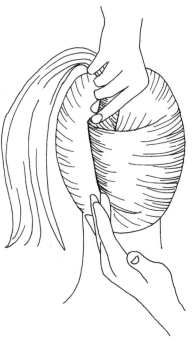

4. Continue loosely twisting the strand until you have reached the ends of the hair.

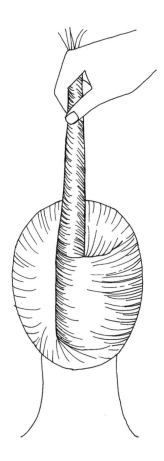

5. Place your left thumb against the head in the crown area.

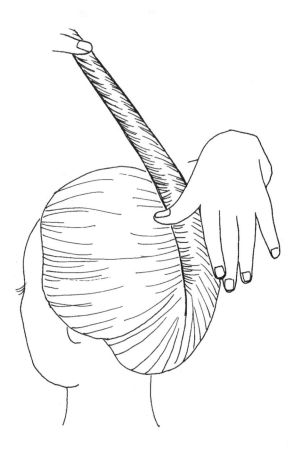

6. Bring the twisted strand down toward the nape and back up again if necessary, so all the hair is folded together.

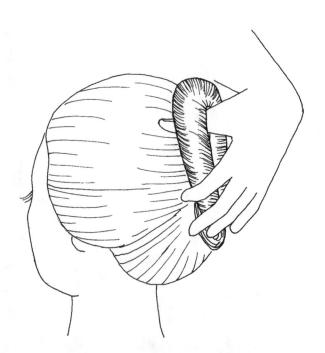

7. Take this folded hair and tuck it under the beginning twist.

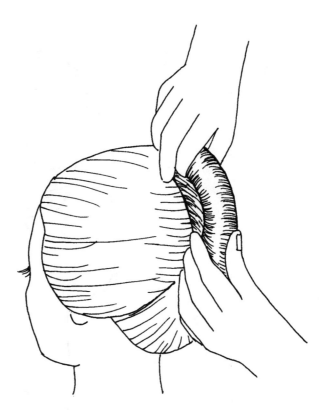

8. Secure along twist with bobby pins and hairpins.

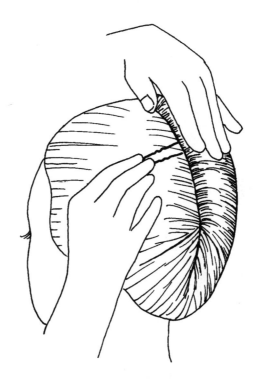

9. The finished style.

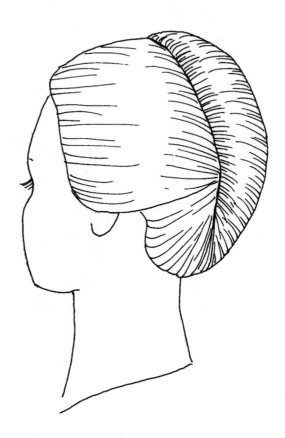

STYLE 18

French Twist with Back-Combing

This technique is for shorter or layered hair that your client wants dressed with a French Twist. You may use a comb or brush to do the backcombing, but whichever you choose, don't pack the backcombing tightly.

Jamie's Law: To create a French Twist as shown, you must follow the numbered section in order.

1. Divide the head into sections as shown.

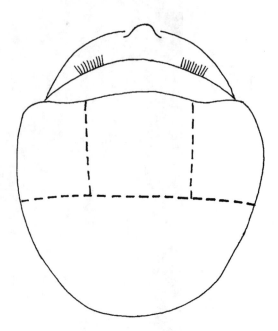

2. Backcomb section 1.

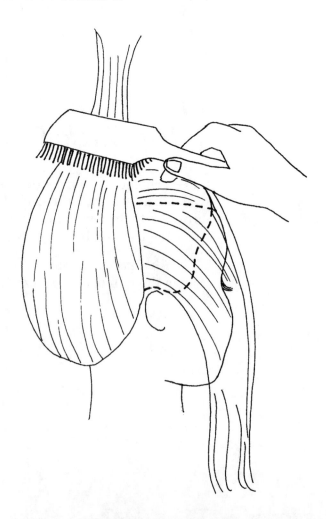

3. Brush all the hair in section #1 over to the right side. Make it as smooth as possible.

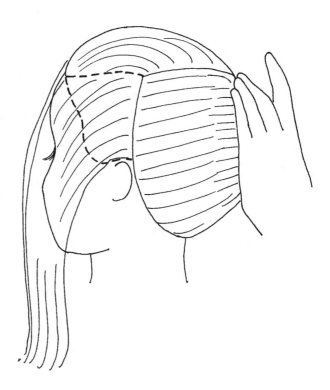

4. Secure hair into this position using bobby pins. Make sure the tips of the bobby pins overlap for a firm hold.

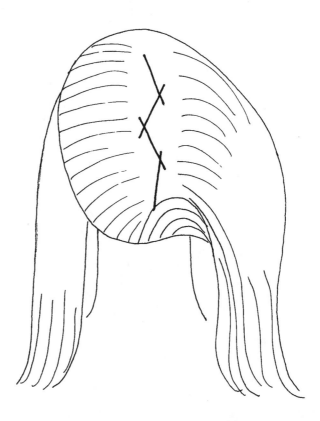

5. Brush the hair to right of bobby pins over to the left. This section will come back over the line of bobby pins. Make as smooth as possible.

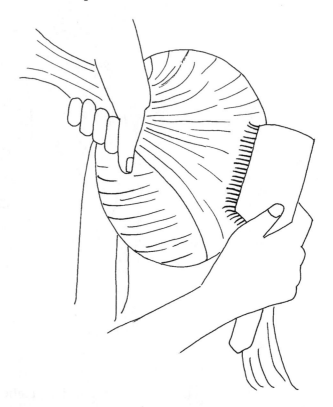

6. Place this section in your right hand, palm facing out, as shown.

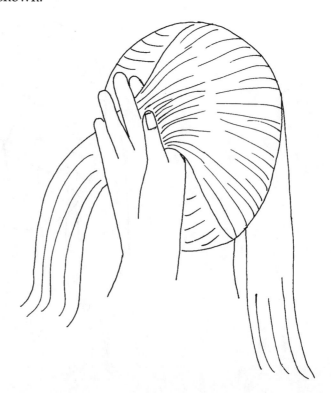

7. Turn hand to the left to face palm against the head. You have made the pleat that forms the twist.

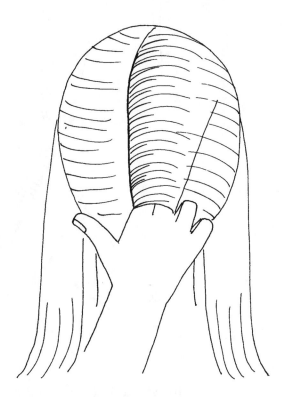

8. Use hairpins to secure the twist.

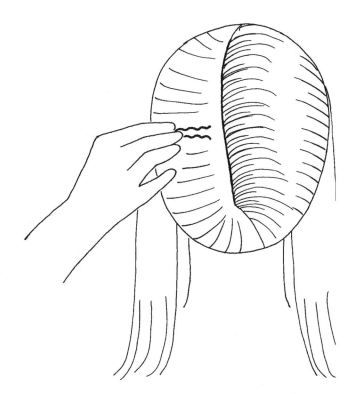

9. Backcomb section 2.

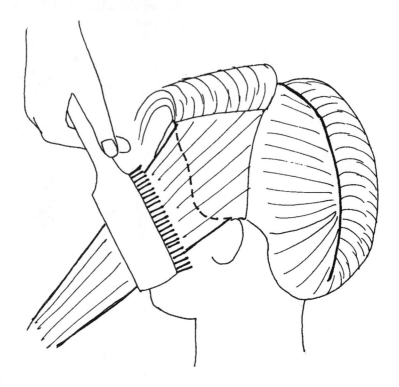

10. Use a brush to smooth out section 2, brushing up into the crown area.

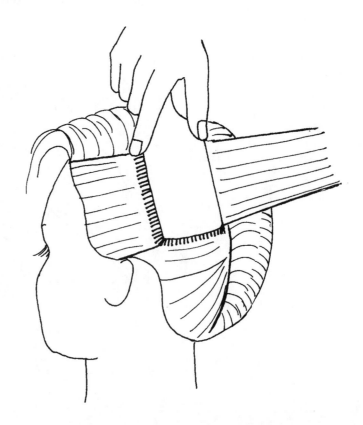

11. Wrap the ends around two fingers of your right hand to make a pincurl.

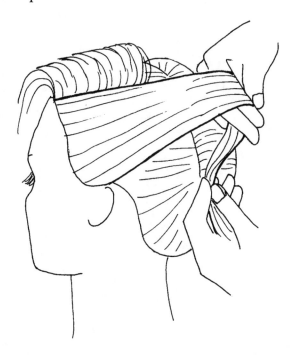

12. Set pincurl into the top of the opening made by the twist. Use bobby pins to secure.

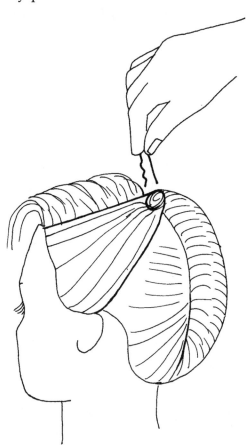

13. Back comb section 3.

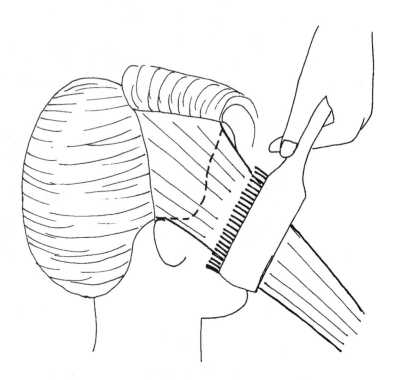

14. Use a brush to smooth out section 3, brushing up into the crown area.

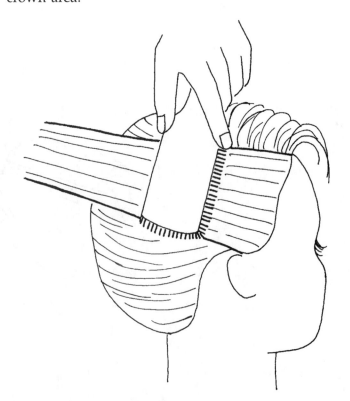

15. Make a pincurl with the ends. Set pincurl into the top of the twist. Make sure the sides are well blended with the previous sections in the back.

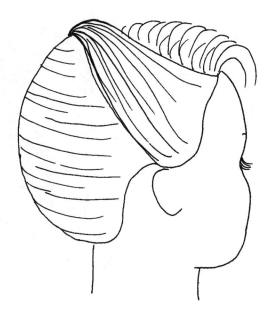

16. Backcomb and smooth out section 4. Make a pincurl and place into the twist to create a smooth finished look. You may need to work with this section of hair more than the others to blend the section together.

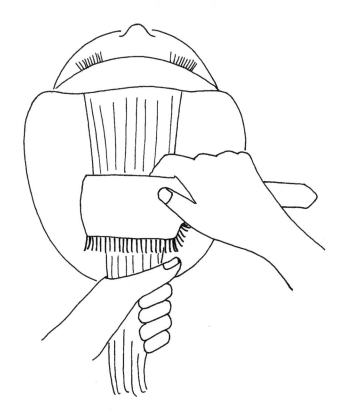

17. When section 4 is smoothly in place it can create a beautiful overlap effect.

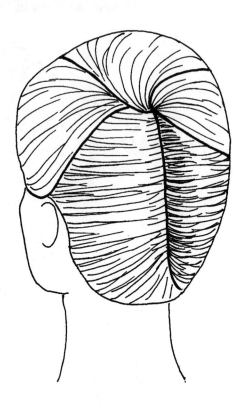

STYLE 19

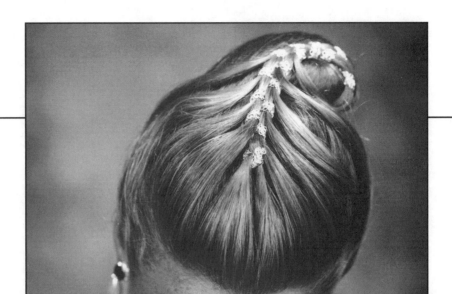

Ribbon Braid with a French Twist

This style is a combination of two different styles previously done. It is a wonderful way to create fullness around the face and accessorize with ribbon at the same time. If you have mastered the 2-Strand Ribbon Braid and the French Twist, this style will be very easy for you. If not, refer back to the styles for details.

Ribbon Braid with a French Twist is best done on dry, long layered or all one-length hair.

Jamie's Law: Make sure to do the French Twist first and secure only the top to hold it while you finish the Ribbon Braid. If you secure the entire French Twist, you won't be able to tuck the ends of the Ribbon Braid into the twist.

1. Divide the head into two sections as shown. The front section should be 2" of hair all the way around the hairline to the ears on both sides. Begin on the remaining hair in the back section.

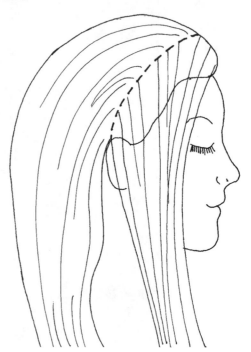

2. Standing in front of your client's right shoulder, comb the hair back into a ponytail and hold it with your left hand, palm facing toward nape with hand in a V position, as shown.

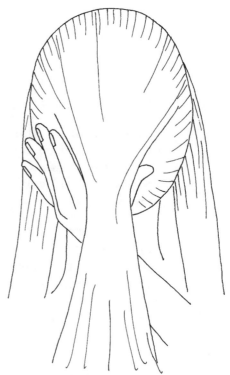

3. Close fingers together making sure to keep hand in the closed "V" position. Do not close hand into a circle as with a ponytail.

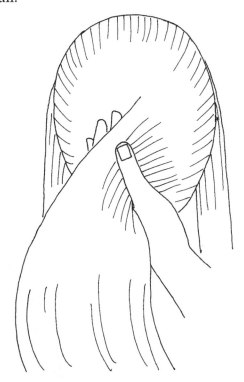

4. Reaching over your client's head with your right arm, grab the hair strand and begin twisting the entire strand to your right.

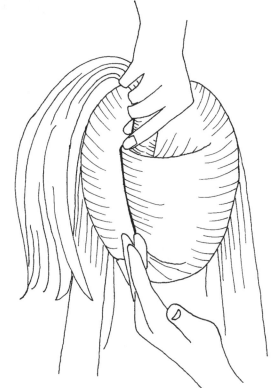

5. Continue loosely twisting the strand until you have reached the ends of the hair.

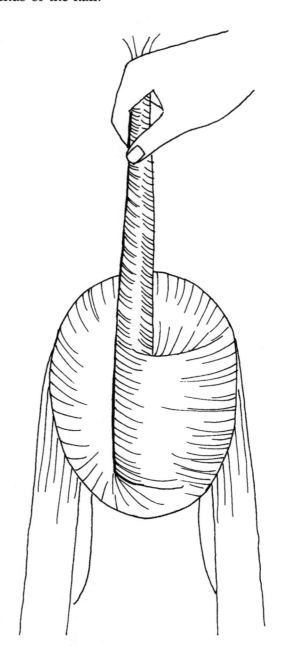

6. Place your left thumb against the head in the crown area.

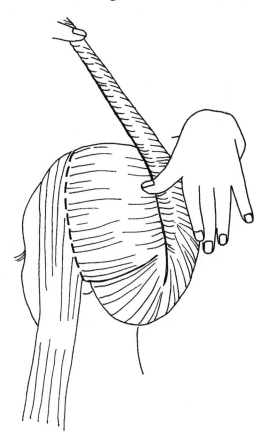

7. Bring the twisted strand down toward the nape and back up again if necessary, so all the hair is folded together.

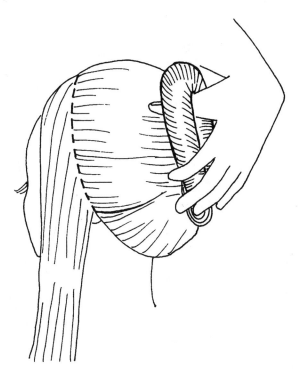

8. Take this folded hair and tuck it under the beginning twist.

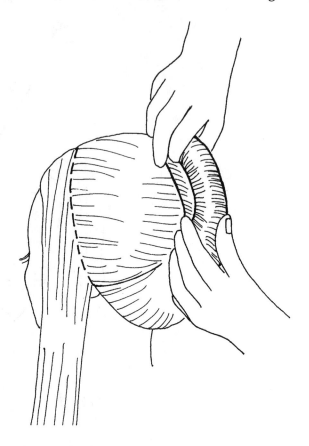

9. Securely pin the top only of the twist as shown. Leave the seam unpinned at this time.

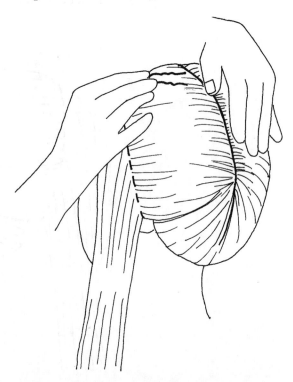

10. Next, do a 2-strand Ribbon Braid on the front section of hair. Take a small section in the bang area, divide into two sections. Tie a ribbon to the left strand.

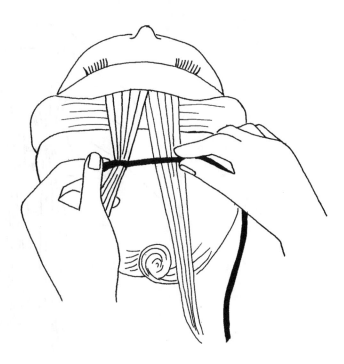

11. While holding the left strand, drop the ribbon down to hang freely.

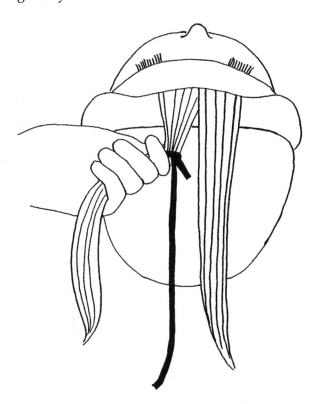

12. Pick up the right strand and place inbetween the index and third fingers, palm up, as shown. Pick up the ribbon with your right hand and bring it under the right strand.

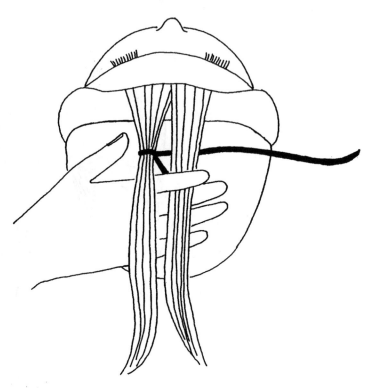

13. Then bring ribbon up and over the right strand. Drop the ribbon to hang freely inbetween the two strands.

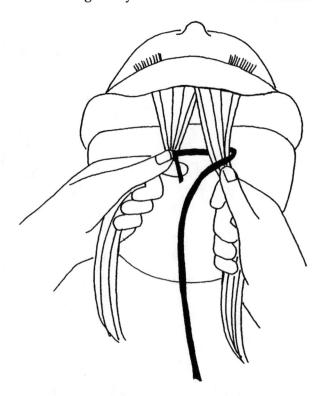

14. Place both strands in your right hand, index finger in-between, palm up, as shown. Allow ribbon to hang freely.

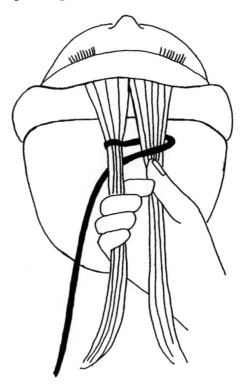

15. Pick up a 1" section on the left side.

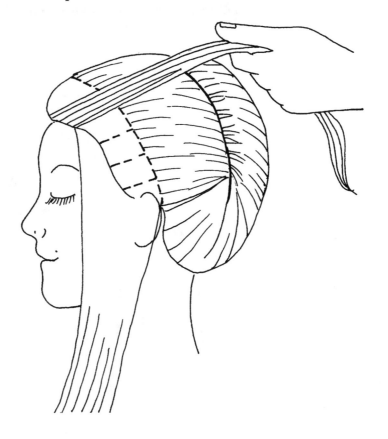

16. Add this section to the left strand already in your hand.

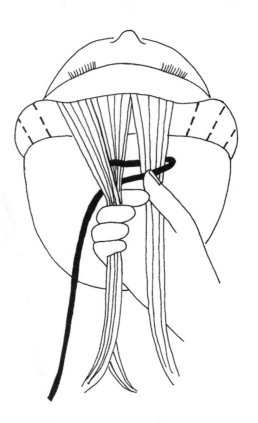

17. Pick up the ribbon with your left hand and bring it under the left strand.

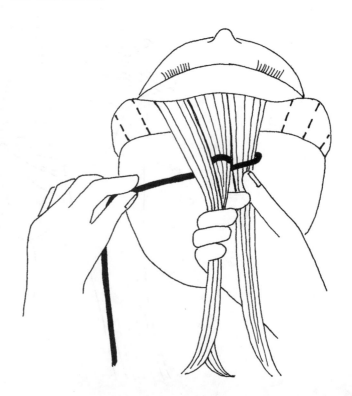

18. Bring ribbon up and over the left strand. Drop the ribbon to hang freely between the two strands.

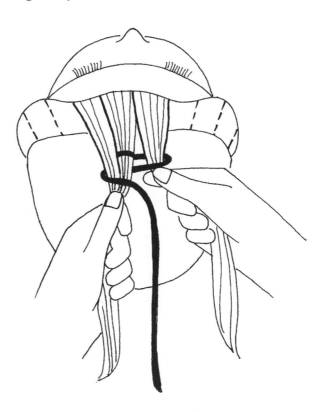

19. Place both strands in your left hand, index finger inbetween, palm up, as shown. Allow ribbon to hang free.

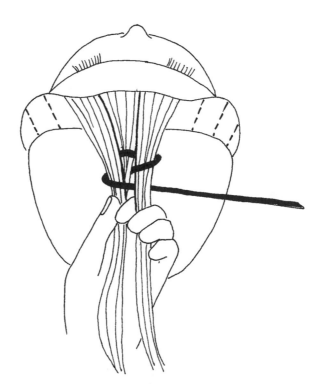

20. Pick up a 1" section on the right side.

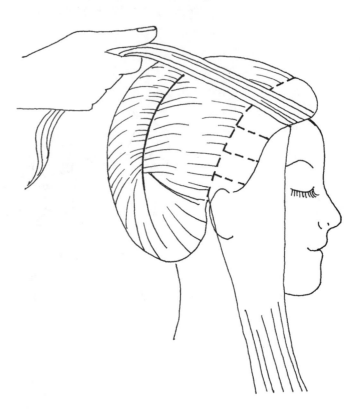

21. Add the section to the right strand already in your hand.

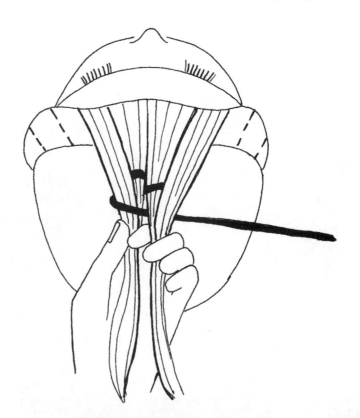

22. Pick up the ribbon with your right hand and bring it under then up and over the right strand. Allow ribbon to hang freely between the two strands.

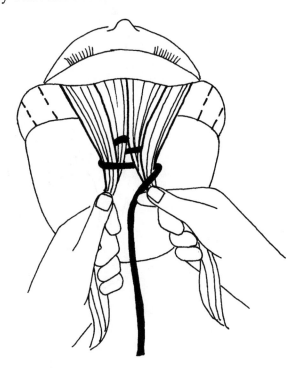

23. Repeat steps 14 through 22 moving down toward the ears with each 1" section picked up. When you run out of sections to pick up, continue doing the figure-eight 5 or 6 more times. Make a loop with the loose ribbon braid as shown.

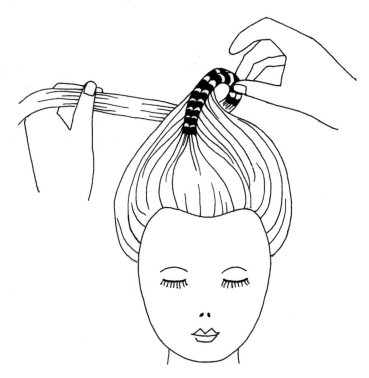

24. Set the loop on top of the French Twist and tuck the free ends under the twist. Pin securely, making sure all ends are tucked under.

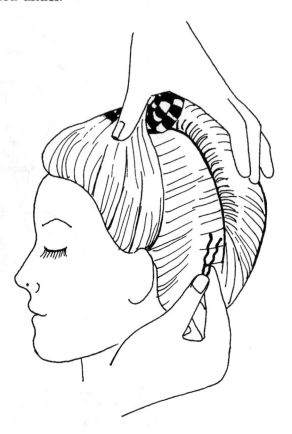

25. It is easy to create fullness by pushing the Ribbon Braid forward, and pinning in that position.

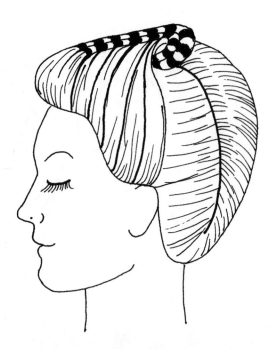

STYLE 20

Overlap Updo

The Overlap Updo looks similar to the Fishtail. The major difference is that this technique calls for backcombing which creates fullness and results in a more formal look. It can be done on dry, all one-length hair as well as dry, long-layered hair.

Jamie's Law: Step 1 is very important to do correctly. The section of hair put into the ponytail serves as the base in which all bobbypins are placed. Do not pin outside the section of hair secured by a rubberband. It could result in the hair slipping out.

1. Section the hair as shown. Make the ponytail base about 2" wide and go from the crown to the nape. Secure with rubberband. This ponytail section will be referred to as the "Ponytail Base" in this style. Next, section out the front from the crown to the hairline in the bang area. Allow all other hair to fall free.

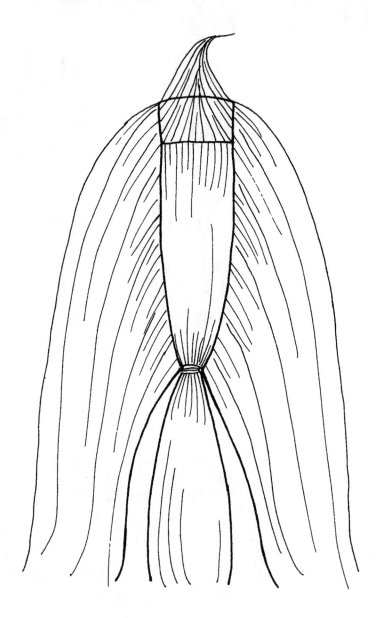

2. Pick up the front bang section.

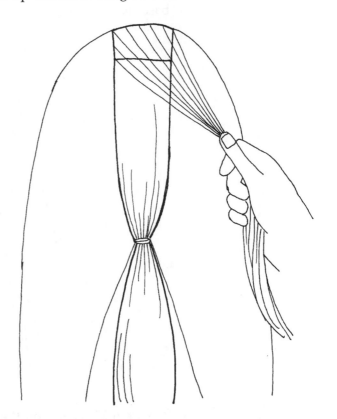

3. Divide the section into two strands and cross the right strand over the left.

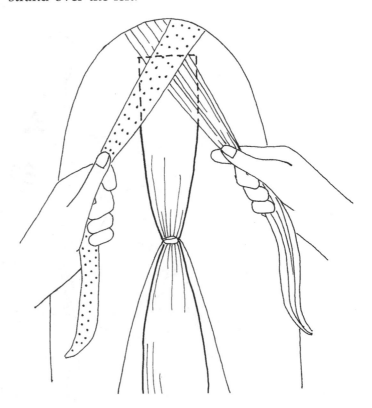

4. Secure the two sections with bobby pins to the ponytail base made in step 1.

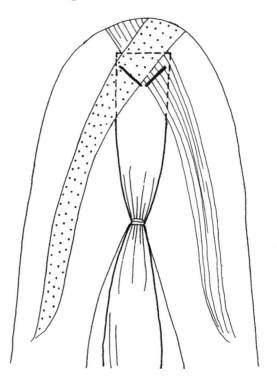

5. Pick up a 2" section on the left side of head. Lightly back-comb this section.

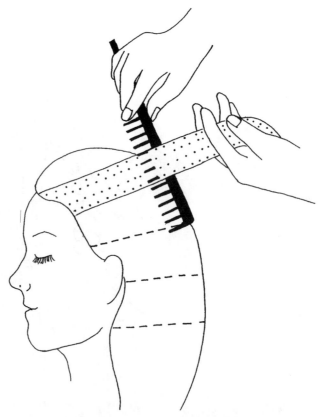

6. Tuck this section underneath the strand on the right you already pinned. Then secure this section with a bobby pin.

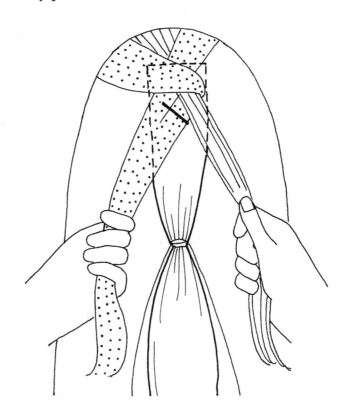

7. Pick up a 2" section on the right side of head. Lightly backcomb this section.

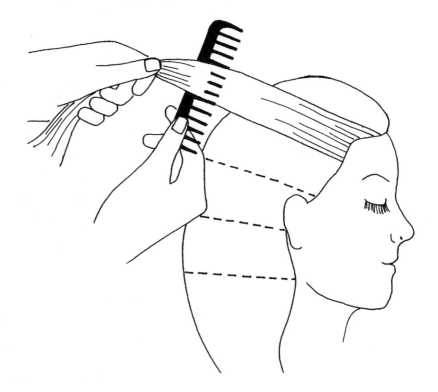

8. Tuck this section underneath the strand on the left that you previously pinned to the ponytail base. Secure this section to the ponytail base.

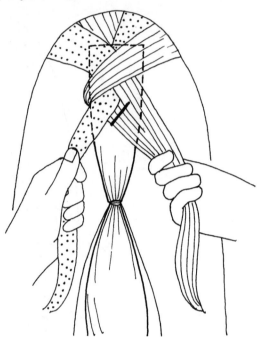

9. Repeat steps 5 through 8, picking up 2" sections as you move down the head. Continue until you reach the nape and run out of sections to pick up. Bend the ends of the ponytail with a curling iron and lightly backcomb for a fuller, free hanging ponytail.

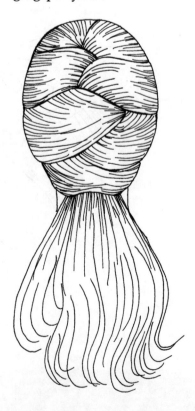

Notes

Notes

Notes

Notes

Notes

Notes

Style.
Savvy.
Solutions.

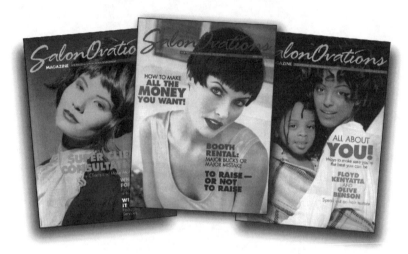

every month.

SalonOvations

SalonOvations is a professional and personal magazine

designed with you in mind. Each issue delivers great

features on personal growth and on-target stories about

the beauty business. Get helpful hints from industry pros

on starting your own salon business and how to satisfy

your clients. Plus, you'll get pages of colorful photos of

the latest trends in haircutting, styling and coloring.

All this at a great price of ~~12~~ **15** issues for only $19.95 a year!

3 FREE issues - Save over 40% (price subject to change)

YES! Send me **3 FREE** issues of *SalonOvations Magazine* plus 12 issues at the special low rate of $19.95! That's a total of 15 issues for the price of 12! – A $33.75 value – **Save over 40%**

Name _____

Signature _____
(order cannot be processed without a signature)

Title _____

Salon or School Name _____

Your Mailing Address _____

City/State/Zip _____

Phone _____

❏ Here's my check or money order for $19.95   ❏ MasterCard   ❏ VISA

Card# _____ Exp Date _____

Job Title: ❏ Student ❏ Hair Colorist ❏ Esthetician ❏ Salon Owner ❏ Teacher/Educator
❏ Hair Stylist ❏ Barber ❏ Nail Technician ❏ Salon Mgr. ❏ Mfr's Rep ❏ Other_____

Type of Business: ❏ School ❏ Full Svc. Salon ❏ Skin Care Salon ❏ Beauty Supply Dist.
❏ Beauty Salon ❏ Nail Salon ❏ Resort or Spa ❏ Manufacturer ❏ Other_____

Clip and mail to: *SalonOvations* Subscriptions, PO Box 10520, Riverton, NJ 08706-8520   code 95013

GUILDFORD **college**

Learning Resource Centre

Please return on or before the last date shown.
No further issues or renewals if any items are overdue.

− 5 JUL 2011
2 1 JAN 2014
2 4 FEB 2015

Class: 646.724 JON
Title: Braids & Updos made easy
Author: Jones, Jamie Rines

WITHDRAWN

151445